NUMEROLOGY FOR BRILLIANCE

Guruchander and Kirn Khalsa

Cover image © Socorro Salazar
Book Design Ram Krishan Singh Khalsa
Illustrations Ram Krishan Kaur Khalsa
Photographs Hargobind Khalsa

Second Edition © 2022 by Purest Potential
ISBN: 979-9867820-4-1

Please Direct all Correspondence and Inquiries to:

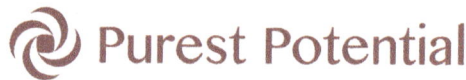

Purest Potential
Santa Fe, NM 87507
www.purestpotential.com

With huge gratitude to all brilliant Kundalini yogis and to our prosperity coach and mentor, John Cundiff, who thrived at life's very edge.

For our yoga family
Stay as close as you can to your own experience
You are the alpha and the omega
Breathe deep and tune in, because all you have to do is
Be You

May all beings be happy, May all beings be at peace
Sat Nam

Our desire is for every person in this world to have an opportunity to master themselves and manifest their Purest Potential.

CONTENTS

THE FUNDAMENTALS

There is One Central Biorhythm from which all of creation, Prakirti, manifests.

Prakirti is highly organized and predictable according to Universal laws.

These laws are observable within and without.

Life requires voltage, prana, and a magnetic field—an aura—to live and Thrive.

Each of the ten bodies needs to pass through the meditative, neutral mind for the soul to achieve liberation.

PRELUDE

It's with great joy and gratitude that we present this information which started way back when...

Thousands of years ago in the East, there were rich Brahmans and there were renunciate yogis. Life dedicated to greater potential, to Spirit, in those times only occurred at the extremes of society. Access to spiritual teachings and experiences was largely available only to those who could afford it, having been born into an upper caste, or those who were willing and often compelled to renounce the entire world. Inner peace only seemed available either deep within the halls of temples or in forest caves and mountaintops. For everyday people, it was incredibly difficult to maintain a sense of peace in the face of the bustling world with its inherent distractions, family and trade. In those times the only option was to leave society, and move to the monastery or the mountain.

Yet, there were spiritual teachers, such as the Buddha and Guru Nanak, who taught that disparities between everyday life and spiritual life were actually non-existent. Every moment they taught, is an opportunity for enlightenment. In this regard, these teachers were no different than any other great spiritual leader or enlightened being. Jesus was a carpenter. Muhammad was a great general. Every great spiritual teacher has been, in his or her own way, a pragmatist. This idea of integration is almost foreign to the Western mind, which considers body, mind, and soul three distinct and separate territories. Worldly concerns are supposedly beneath those of great spiritual caliber. It is almost as if one can be expected to live as a soul alone, without a body or mind. The examples of these teachers suggest that this separation is counterproductive from a spiritual standpoint. If you spend any time studying spiritual teachings, it becomes very clear that enlightenment is not simply the process of removing the influence of the world on you, but also involves taking the experience of enlightenment and sharing it with others. With this two-fold intention, our journey starts.

SO WHAT ABOUT YOU?

There are plenty of yoga and meditation classes you can attend, countless religious ceremonies in which you can participate, and a myriad of ways for you to give money or help others. But what does it mean to do any of these? With so many options, how do you choose what to do? How can you know the course, or which practice is the most effective one for you to do? How are you supposed to understand the volumes and volumes of, sometimes conflicting, information about what you are here to be and manifest?

The aim of this book is to help you answer these questions and to provide a factual and grounded approach to understanding seemingly disparate teachings on a wide variety of subjects—all of which pertain in some way to your spiritual development, your brilliance. We offer you a great amount of detail about yogic philosophy and esoteric traditions, and at the center of it all we will highlight the awareness you hold being in-body. As has been shown by the lives of various spiritual teachers, the process of living includes your active, in-body participation with the world around you. So, our journey begins with your biology using your own experiences and finding clarity from your senses—from what you can see, feel, taste, touch and smell. You will find that by practicing the methods obtained through the study of yoga and energy healing modalities, that your body and it's many aspects will awaken and connect to more subtle systems. In turn, these subtle connections will enable you to gain a deeper experience of the Self.

Our premise is that there is no negative imagery at all involved with this system. Life is a set of circumstances, which unfold and teaches us that all wisdom and events are beyond anything negative, when used to generate more awareness. Everything that happens is designed to offer an opportunity to make a choice about what direction we want to move into. Without darkness

3

there would be no light and it is your choice where you want to dwell. "Guilt is optional" on this journey.

CHANGE MUST HAPPEN

The process for Purest Potential takes place when we choose to learn from our interactions with the polarities and shift our individual awareness to group awareness, and then to universal awareness. Most of us would rather skip the whole group awareness experience because it is in our relationship to the other where our buttons really get pushed and our opportunities for transformation show up most often and most clearly! We know because we lived in ashrams for decades, where it was never certain that your lunch would still be in the fridge when you got home.

Group living provides the opportunity to see beyond the obvious, to observe the deeper process of transformation, to not get bent out of shape over those things which ultimately don't matter, to stay committed and clear on why we practice, which is to live as yogis, unaffected by the play of the opposites and then to serve.

SO, JUST HOW DO WE PROPOSE TO DO THIS?

With this clear intent:

- Master your 10 bodies
- Live from the sacred space of the 11th embodiment
- Serve

It is when being mindful of your potential, that you develop the flexibility to use all parts of the psyche. There are ten parts of the psyche: one physical Body, three mental Bodies and six subtle Bodies. This system acknowledges that everyone has the same potential, that there are no superior beings, and we are all One on this journey to manifest our soul's brilliance.

And this is just how brilliant you are:

You have a soul, three parts of your mind and a physical body. The third eye, the arc line, is the balance point between your physical existence and your spiritual existence. From your 7th chakra, the 10th gate, rays of light shoot out which surround your physical body in a 9-foot sphere. This flow creates the electromagnetic field around the body, the aura. When all contractions and polarities in the first 5 chakras are neutralized, this aura becomes nine feet wide and creates a sphere of eighteen feet in diameter. With this extended aura intact, you then have the ability to channel the universal life force, prana, into your physical existence through the Pranic Body. Then your Pranic Body automatically recharges your subtle body system from the connection to an infinite supply of energy....

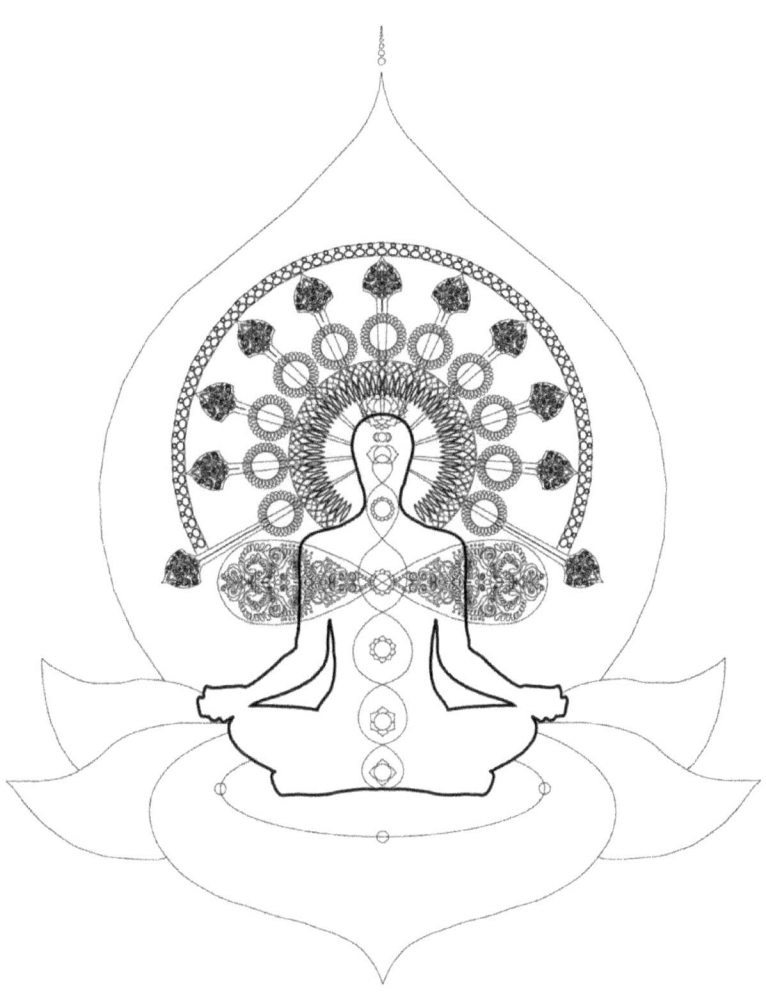

We studied many books to find the patterns, which other cultures had observed, in order to recognize where dis-harmony came from. We found charts describing the energetic patterns of health and dis-ease, of expansion and contraction, in books on Chinese medicine, Ayurveda, macrobiotics and in the Touch For Health courses. It was interesting to notice that these charts presented many similarities to the kundalini yoga teachings. We realized that there had to be one energy pattern that flows through all beings and that this was described in many different ways, yet it was the same electrical system at the causal level. This is the concept that we will explore in our book.

In the end, you will have a kind of schematic diagram for what we call your "Purest Potential" (a collection of functional ways of seeing) that when practiced will increase your awareness, making an incredibly large amount of data available to you at any given moment. This will allow you the opportunity to make more informed choices that can lead to happiness, health, prosperity and a life that expresses your Purest Potential.

* **Purest** is clear and true; without any discordant quality

***Potential** is that which you are capable of being or becoming

As we always say, prosperity means a pro-spirit life. Your unique spirit has so many ways of expressing itself—and how to experience them is what this book will enlighten you with. Brilliance...

Chapter 1
PUREST POTENTIAL

The kundalini lifestyle started to hone our awareness to the subtle energies that are tied into the body and calibrated to raise individual awareness. In 1979 we were also students of Chiropractic, Chinese Medicine, Applied Kinesiology, Radionics, and Ayurvedic healing. In other words, we had a lot to assimilate. We studied and practiced as we sought out how best to understand the validity and interrelation of these various systems. Since then, our healing business and yoga center have grown and thrived and the daily application by students and patients of these systems has provided feedback. We have seen firsthand that the chakras and the Ten Bodies have a very special relationship.

What follows is Guruchander's exploration of this relationship between the chakras and the Ten Bodies.

Here is the original question I sat with: Do the chakras correspond to the Ten Bodies? From my meditative inquiry and practice I realized that chakras have their action and reaction and the Ten Bodies have their action and reaction. They are different sets of equipment and the implication of observing them in this way is a promising avenue for discovery and ultimately Self Mastery.

At a yoga course in 1981, we spent nearly the entire time focused on the sixth Chakra and, the "arc line". We did many special meditations for the Sixth Chakra which allowed us to experience that the effect of the harmonized Body, the arc line, of the sixth Chakra was the key to personal strength. We perceived the sixth Body, the arc line, to be the most concentrated part of the electromagnetic energy which "binds" the rest of our energies together by way of this arc line.

The experience of the arc line in that meditation course altered my frame of reference for looking at the possibilities of the connections between the Chakras and the Bodies. What I then realized was that the chakra is a location where two meridians intersect. That the electric interaction from one positively charged and one negatively charged meridian creates a magnetic field. This field is what holds the knowledge of that interaction, and this is what we call the Body. The chakra is an electric location, and the body is a magnetic field created by this electric interaction.

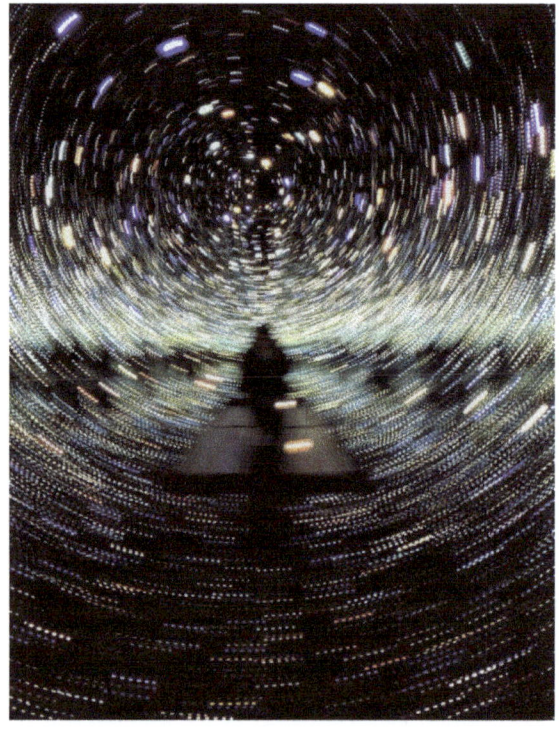

Numerology for Brilliance - is a blueprint for the body, mind, and the first layers of subtle energy. What is outlined is a complete map for how any person can operate at their fullest potential. Having an understanding of the association between the first seven chakras and first seven bodies opens access to another realm of understanding—one that deepens the connection between chakras and the psyche, and this 'applied awareness' facilitates the expression of your Purest Potential.

OUR PROMISE
Purest Potential provides a system for you to hold your life with more awareness and courage.

OUR REQUEST
In order to participate with Purest Potential we ask that you commit to:
- Live as a "self sensory being".
- Engage with a "learning community".
- Share this information with others.

THE POTENTIAL
When you stand in your power of choice you can claim a better future for yourself, your loved ones, and the global community.

COMMUNITY
For individual consciousness to be sustainable and actualized, we need a community that is committed to learn and grow together, a community where each person is accountable for their own process (self sensory) and allowed to make mistakes, a community that provides space for self-reflection and encouragement, a learning community! The only mistake, which is not encouraged, is the same one.
What follows is Kirn's exploration on conscious community.

I found that the typical purpose for community are based on those who:

- Share the same interest.
- Want to bring about change.

- Live in the same location.
- Do the same things.
- Are brought together by external events.

My observation was that these traditional models were either based on circumstances or action and I longed for a deeper, more sustainable community. When I was much younger, I had the same longing for a more profound way to exercise. Then, when I was fifteen I found my answer in kundalini yoga. My search for conscious community however, took a lot longer.

Fast forward to 2010, we are at a party, packed to the gills, in Santa Fe and were introduced to John Cundiff, a fortune 500 coach. Within minutes of meeting he said to me, "Well, you are a control freak aren't you?" This got my attention, as this is not the way proper people behave at a perfectly nice party. I, of course, said, "Yes!" We exchanged business cards, which thankfully I had on me, and said our goodbyes. I received a phone call 5 days later from John. He asked if we would mentor with him, he had a feeling that there was a greater reason for our meeting. It turns out that John had been diagnosed with cancer and wanted to share his coaching process with a community other than the business world.

What I realized after some time was that John had re-discovered a Yogic model for prosperity. The Purushartha system, which is based on: amplifying inner strengths, redirecting inherent weaknesses, a commitment to higher learning, and encouraging each other's known potential.

The traditional application of this method is to assign the 4 aspects of manifestation as goals for living:

- Moksha - Liberation
- Kama - Pleasure
- Dharma – Duty
- Artha -Wealth

In chapter 8 you will learn how to apply the Purushartha system as the bridge to move from the Self-sensory personal experience into community.

Personal: The discovery that you "live" inherently from one of those quadrants and need to become accountable for your contribution.

Community: Where you engage from your core contribution with a community committed to learning how to manifest Purest Potential for each other and the community.

The most important aspect of this whole journey is to be exactly who you came here to be!

Throughout this book, you will discover the brilliance and compassion of the Purest Potential method, a way to observe and share your essential gifts.....just keep reading!

PRACTICE
Pushma Kriya: Flower Meditation

To take you out of self-limiting mental processes and to experience your potential.

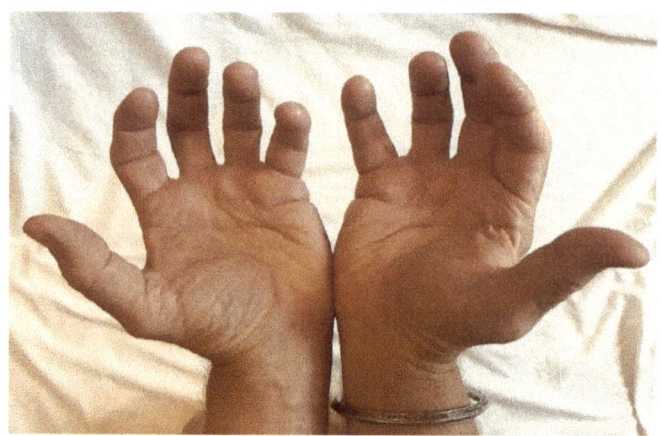

1) Open hands like flowers and make tiger claws with fingers, like in Kung Fu. Curve fingers and thumbs, and keep separated by 1 inch each. Keep fingers TIGHT.

Mudra sits 10 inches our from heart center, palms face up.

Press only the pinky edges of hands above the wrists together and leave one inch between the mounds of the pinky fingers, while pressing the bottom part firmly together.

2) Close eyes and visualize flowers and colors at the forehead, hold this mudra for 7 minutes. Then, relax the mudra into your lap and meditate. Float and float beyond the stars, the sun and moon, and into an infinite world. Experience your little 'I am' and the infinite 'I am' at the same time.

Summary of the Purest Potential Process:

- Become a self-sensory being who can control the reactivity of the first five bodies (corresponding to the first five chakras) and consciously create a state of balance, which encourages the kundalini to rise.

- Master the 6th body (the ajna chakra), and expand the following subtle bodies.

- Strengthen the 7th body (the aura), to contain and protect the balanced manifestation of the first six bodies. Then with continued practice, the volume of magnetic potency in the 7th body increases and that allows your 9th and 10th bodies to radiate at full potential.

- Create a maximum radiation in the magnetic field of the 8th body (the pranic body), which then directs more prana into the self-contained system of the 7th body.

- Radiate the Etheric Body of the 9th and the circumvent force of the 10th body at full potential.

- Manage all 10 Bodies through the 11th Embodiment.

- Be 100% accountable for your Purushartha contribution.

- Participate in a learning community.

- Serve.

The possibility for Purest Potential is based on a self-sensory human who is aware of their subtle anatomy and committed to share this experience for the greater good.

Chapter 2
ESSENTIALS FOR THE SELF-SENSORY BEING

Lord Vishnu was up in the heavens—completely bored with the perfection of it all. To shake life up a bit, he decides to go down to Earth to try out living a worldly life. So he chooses to become a mother pig and pretty soon because of all the little piglets and demands of earthly living, Vishnu becomes more and more oblivious of his true nature. The other gods have been watching this, and they become concerned that Vishnu might never return to heaven. They decide to come down to earth to remind Vishnu of his true nature. It took a lot of convincing because the mirage of maya had Vishnu in a state of amnesia, believing that he was in fact a mama pig.

Sounds familiar? How often do we have to shake ourselves out of thinking that our true, unbounded nature is something mysterious and impossible to attain.

The essentials for the self-sensory being described in this chapter are a 'way of life', a means to manifest your brilliance, your unbounded nature. A self-sensory being is sovereign unto themselves, their own guru. A self-sensory being has learned how to observe their own energy, and how to correct to a state of balance. This way of life is best supported with the following four essentials:

1) **Sankalpa** – intention.

2) **Pratyahar** - the process of directing your mind towards Infinity.

3) **Dharma** - that which upholds and supports your purpose in life and <u>Karma</u> - the blocks that impede the process of living your dharma.

4) **Shunia** - the still point which facilitates the state of Saibhang - Self-initiation.

SANKALPA - THE INTENTION
The first essential for the self-sensory being.

Where we declare our intention

Various systems will be discussed throughout this book to offer you information and strategies, which we hope you will apply to your life with enthusiasm. Having a clear personal intention and stating exactly why you want to make all this effort—why it matters to you—will ground you so that you're not swept up in the rush of new information. Moving forward, you will be able to ask yourself the liberating questions necessary for personal growth and even brilliant enlightenment. Enlightenment is a word that stands for an experience. It is an experience everyone wants because of the promise that comes with it, health and happiness. We do not promise any specific results. However, the guide provided in chapters 5, 6 and 7 is a tool to assist in attenuating you to a brilliant life. Clarifying your intention, our first essential, is what starts the process.

We invite you to sit down and examine how familiar you are with your life's intention. Your potential will not be realized by asking what and how, but by asking who and why. Don't worry if the answer isn't immediately apparent. Take your time as you incorporate the following pranayam (breath technique) and take personal inventory.

PRACTICE

Sit up straight and close the eyes.

Inhale in 4 parts, exhale in 1 smooth breath through the nose.

Continue this pranayam and after 1-minute start to mentally add the mantra 'Sa' 'Ta' 'Na' 'Ma" on each of the four segments of the inhalation and smoothly add the mantra 'Wahe Guru' to the exhalation.

Continue this pranayam powerfully, for at least 3 minutes, combining the force of the breath with the power of the navel (pumping with each breath) as this will allow the prana to open up your chakras. To finish, inhale and suspend the breath. Exhale and continue with the questions below.

*To get you started: *remember that this journey is more about awareness and less about analyzing, so keep breathing. Inhale belly out, exhale belly in, and keep breathing long and deep.*

When I die what do I want people to remember about the kind of person I was? (your who)

What do I feel passionate about? (your why)

Holding what you just wrote in your awareness, do the following pranayam to connect to your essence. This one works so fast that you will only do it for a total of 3 breaths.

Connect the tips of the thumbs with the tips of the index finger and cross your hands just above the wrists, with both palms facing the heart. Hold this mudra touching your heart. Inhale deeply and exhale completely. While holding the breath out, mentally chant the following mantra while pumping the navel on each word (21 pumps total).

> *Haree haree haree haree haree haree har*
> *Haree haree haree haree haree haree har*
> *Haree haree haree haree haree haree har*

Mentally chant and pump the navel with the breath held out for a total of 3 breaths.

Sit for a few minutes, opening up to your essential nature.

Reread what you wrote for your why and who and complete the box below.

My Sankalpa – My Intention

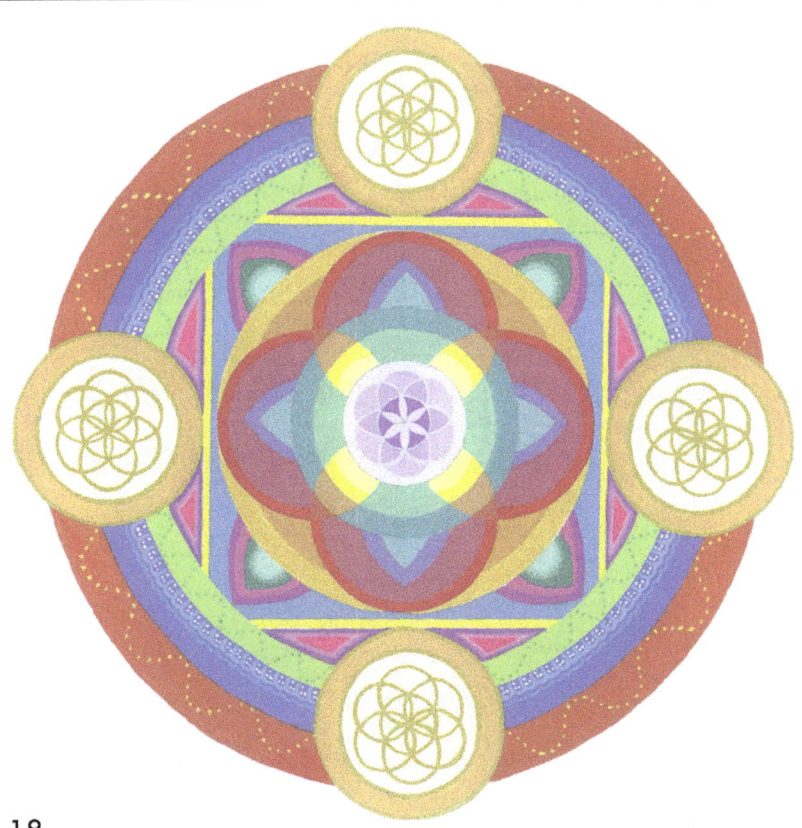

PRATYAHAR – Dedicated Devotion
The second essential for the self-sensory being

Where we engage with what matters

With a clear intention the next essential is the practice of pratyahar, the science of dedicated devotion. It occurs when you can synchronize your mind toward the Infinite, holding a conscious awareness of the Sacred. This is what allows you to 'sense' where to engage. When you are synchronized toward that which is beyond time and space, beyond the polarities, then, you can engage with what matters, your intention!

This much overlooked and misunderstood yoga practice is one of the 8 limbs of yoga. Reflect on this fact that Patanjali Rishi* named pratyahar as one of the eight limbs of yoga. This indicates that it is as important as asana, pranayama and deep meditation! Pratyahar happens when synchronizing (or contracting) all your energies into the awareness of the Infinite—beyond polarities, ego and the polarized fluctuations of the mind.

Now, you may have already observed that living in a state of pratyahar can feel like a double-edged sword because as you engage with your intention, you begin to notice all the times where you align with your drama instead.

How do yogis support the state of pratyahar and live consistently beyond the polarities of the mind? Here are some practices:

- Be in nature to decrease influence from media and phones.
- Burn incense or ghee lamps.
- Use of an altar.
- Practice Puja*.
- Visualization.
- Food fast.
- Cold shower, ishnaan*.
- Observe silence.

Pratyahar becomes possible when we meditate, practice our asanas, visit sacred places, and burn incense and ghee lamps. We find it in the company of the sadhus and, by offering our actions to the Divine, at altars all around our homes and gardens.

Pratyahar can infuse all the choices you make to remember infinity is your identity in your everyday life. Pratyahar is how your yoga moves off the mat. A conscious lifestyle based on daily habits, informed by pratyahar, is how we manifest our intention.

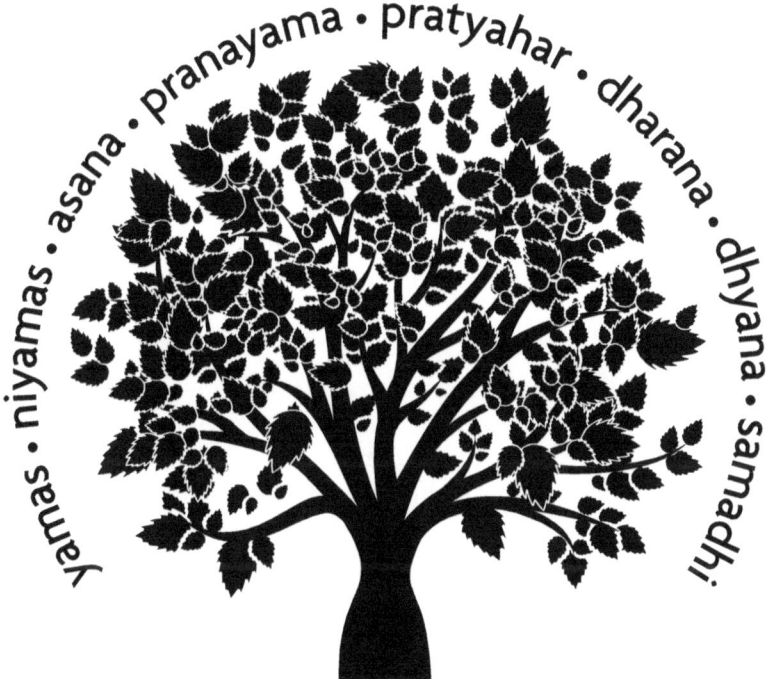

yamas · niyamas · asana · pranayama · pratyahar · dharana · dhyana · samadhi

8 Limbs of Yoga

Pratyahar Illuminates
- what you eat.
- what you drink.
- where you shop.

- the company you keep.
- how you dress.
- where you invest your money.
- how you speak.
- what music you listen to.
- what pictures you have in your house.
- what car you drive.
- and so much more.....all with great enthusiasm!

You can do your practice with the intention to get rocks and you will get rocks, or you can do your practice with the intention to receive diamonds and you will receive diamonds. The choice is yours. Let your clear intention be a diamond and let pratyahar orient your lifestyle towards that diamond; otherwise, it won't remain with you long term. Pratyahar protects you from both the fluctuations of your own mind and the pressures to conform to what's popular in the world around you. It's because of Pratyahar, that your intention becomes your lived experience.

Let's take a yoga break as you consider: "Do I engage my energy to manifest my Intention?"

Here is a simple asana to get your energy flowing: spine flexes. Sit in easy pose and hold on to your shins with both hands. Now, hold the head fairly level and inhale as you move the spine forward with a gentle pull on the shins. Exhale as you round your spine backwards. Continue this smooth movement with a strong breath. After 3 minutes you will be ready to complete the next inquiries:

I shop for most of my food at: _____

I invest my earnings in: _____

I donate ___% to _____charity each month

The car I drive supports, does not support my commitment to living sustainably.

When I get sick I most often see an MD, Chiropractor, or

I visit nature and reduce the influence from media, and from my phone _____times per week.

I visit sacred sites _____ per month.

I burn incense, candles, ghee lamps, or sage to clear my space _____ per week.

I enjoy silence _____ times per week.

I connect with the divine daily through prayer, dance, art or play _____ times per week.

I keep the company of people who are kind and spiritual.

I feed my body healthy, alive, nutritious and tasty food 3 meals a day, 2 meals a day, _____

Other :

My Sankalpa is:

Reflect on your answers and observe where you can make some adjustments, so that your lifestyle can better support and express your intention.

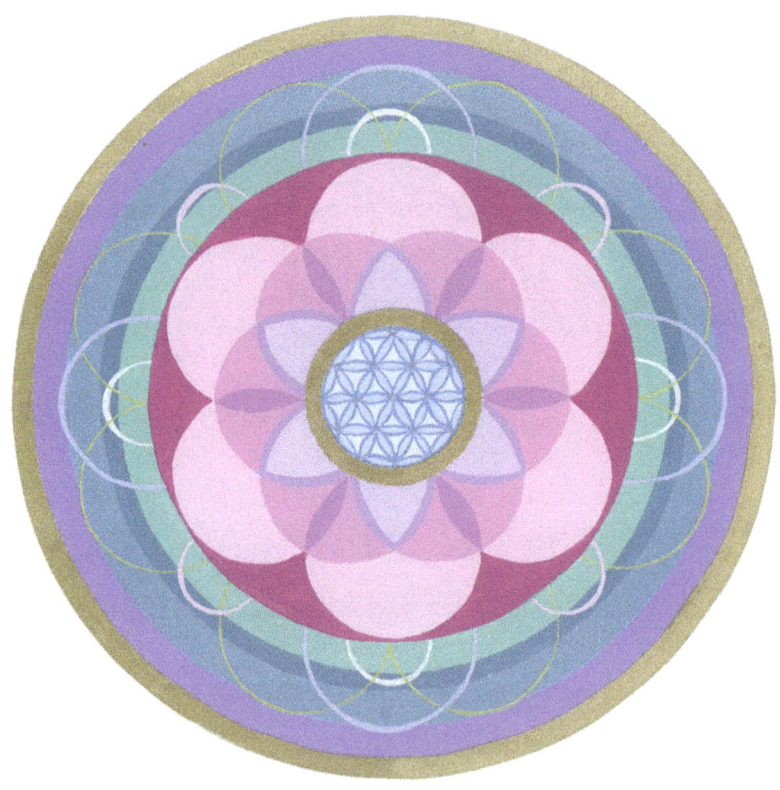

DHARMA & KARMA
The third essential for the Self-sensory being

Where we get to make it real

With a clear intention and the promise of engaging with what matters, the next essential step is how we make our intention real. The word dharma means that which upholds and supports your "purpose in life." Dharma has both a personal and universal application: Personally it is how you manifest your unique purpose, it is the road which carries you. Karma is also the universal law through which we all get to learn from our actions. Consider these dynamics in the light of your newly examined intention. These applications suggest a microcosmic and macrocosmic view of life that is best lived when the two match. The universal law of Dharma is observed through the law of Karma. When your actions are aligned with the universal law of Dharma (conscious action) there is no karma (reaction). When you experience karma, it is an indication that you are out of alignment with the universal laws of Dharma.

With an objective observation, you can clearly see that the Self Sensory path is not the easiest road to travel. Adding this notion to the confusion that an expanding consciousness can cause, it is easy to see that your Dharma can become less than clear. You will notice that with more awareness of your potential, at any given moment and at any given point along your path, you have exactly everything you need. It may not look like what you wanted, but it is exactly what you need to "level up." Basically, once you adopt a dharmic outlook, you will be able to hold on to your vision and have the patience to trust and let it unfold for you. Over time, you will notice that connecting your dharma with your intention is much like learning a foreign language. It isn't always easy or familiar. We encourage you to find the joy in the process and not to fall prey to the endless opportunities of self-criticism that this journey offers. In other words, honor and, most importantly, DEFINE the road that carries you.

KARMA

The beauty of taking the approach of self-awareness is that there is no hidden agenda. At first glance, it may seem unattractive with the accountability it entails. The opposite of dharma is karma. Karma, a word with many connotations, essentially means the blocks that impede the process of living your dharma. Karma refers to actions that are not completed. As long as our actions still hold a polarity frequency—positive or negative— they have not been integrated consciously to neutrality. This 'charge' is the roadblock to manifest your dharma.

Karma however has nothing to do with blame. I once saw a mother trying to "control" her child who was running around for the sheer joy of it all and happened to fall down. The mother scolded, "See, that is your bad karma for not listening to me." Ouch, that hurt me just hearing it! To put a paradigm of shame, guilt and fear on top of a universal law, which is available to bring greater awareness, simply misses the point.

When you create the right relationship with karma, you will notice that you live with greater self-awareness. As you commit to live within your dharma, karma must present itself! Have you noticed that as soon as you commit to your destiny, it seems that all the land mines go off? This is when a lot of unseasoned spiritual travelers say to themselves, "See, I am not supposed to do this because it is too hard ... it is just not meant to be ... it couldn't be God's will because it is so hard." The seasoned travelers however, know that the land mines are a very important part of the journey. They are what remind us to reorient towards the frequency of the soul's purpose, our Dharma.

PRACTICE to overcome reactivity and re-orient to dharma:

Sat Kriya: A fundamental kriya to Kundalini Yoga, it directly stimulates and channels the kundalini energy to move up the sushmana channel. Sit on the heels and lift your arms up with palms together. Interlace all fingers except your index fingers, which point up. Those who identify masculine, cross the right thumb over the left thumb and those who identify feminine cross the left thumb over the right. As you pull in your navel, chant "Sat" powerfully and chant "Nam" as you relax the navel. To end, inhale and apply MB, then exhale and hold your breath out as you apply Maha Bandh (all locks) and visualize the energy moving out of the tenth gate (top of your head) into the Cosmos. Inhale and relax with your forehead on the ground. **Practice 3 – 31+ minutes.**

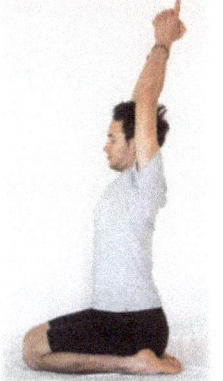

Generate some tapasia (psychic heat) right now so you can open up to subtle expressions of prana. This will change the caliber of your nervous system, so you can enjoy the subtler frequencies of the higher chakras and re-orient to your Dharma.

Karmic Challenges are essential to growth and come to us at all times on the Self-awareness journey. With a mindfulness practice the way in which we react to those challenges begins to change. We see this when we watch a baby getting ready to walk. She will perform triangle pose for preparation; it's a sure bet that she will fall, but no baby has ever given up on the urge to walk because she got discouraged from all the falling. At that wise young age she knows that struggle and falling down are part of learning to walk life's good road.

Instead of living life with judgment about your karmic lessons, we are offering a guide that highlights the areas where you need more balance. At every stage we encourage you to move from self-criticism to self-awareness. The challenges along the way are not because you did something wrong and now you have to deal with the bad karma you incurred. Karma is not good or bad—

it is only that which is not completely processed through the neutrality of the fourth chakra, the sacred heart. Yogis see karma as a signpost along the road to awareness. Some signs tell us to slow down and others tell us to turn left or right. Our choice is always to ignore the signs or to pay attention.

We encourage you to pay attention and increase your sensitivity so that you can notice the signs early on and make the adjustments. You know the story: first, you get a reminder that is similar to getting a tap on the shoulder and then, perhaps a kick in the shins. If you still choose to ignore the signs, then the proverbial truck will hit you. We all signed up for the same journey—to live liberated from the polarities of life. You can do it now or later; it's your choice. The earlier you 'get' the message, the easier the course correction is likely to be. Contrary to the popular belief that ignorance is bliss, we have found that ignorance is actually painful—physically, emotionally and spiritually.

Karma presents itself in any number of ways, but is always recognizable by the intensity of resistance it offers. Again, bringing these metaphysical terms down to earth and considering your life's potential, look at the things that have prevented you from achieving it so far. Don't feel intimidated or overwhelmed. Simply pay attention to that which causes you mental and emotional turmoil, merely by thinking about it; and you will have located your karmic blocks.

Let's connect with the belly now as we root into our bodies and connect to our third chakra, the navel center. Ask the question, "What are the karmic blocks which prevent me from living my purest potential?" With this process, you will get in touch with your shadow side—the side that is not committed to your healthy progress and often throws up roadblocks.

PRACTICE

To begin the meditation, sit tall and close your eyes. Extend your arms straight out to the sides parallel to the earth, make fists with the hands and point the index fingers out with palms facing down.

Inhale through the mouth through a rolled tongue, (if you cannot roll your tongue just make an O with your mouth and lay your tongue on the lower lip) and exhale through the nose. Do this cooling breath, called Sitali Pranayam, for at least 3 minutes and up to 11 minutes.

When you complete the meditation, please sit for a few minutes and allow clarity around the answer to emerge for you, and then write.

My karmic blocks: what would I rather not have anyone know about me?

An example, some women learn that by being flirtatious they can get energy from men. However when a flirtatious woman starts her spiritual journey the mindfulness practices bring this shadow side to light and she observes that the focus of her mind is either to flirt or to be alert. The mind however cannot serve two masters; it is either alert and serves the soul, or it flirts and serves the ego. So how then do we change these deep karmic lessons?

You cannot think or wish yourself into a different state, because the mind can't heal the mind. Instead, with a karmic, deeply repetitive pattern it is necessary to change the actual energetic patterns, similar to breaking an addiction. The healing practices described in this book focus on changing these karmic energetic patterns. In this new age, awareness is what heals. So don't rush this part of your process. You need the daily structure in your life to create greater sensitivity, the clarity around what makes you - You, and the awareness of how that expresses itself. This is where the rubber meets the road, where you get to make it all real.

My daily structure on the road that carries me includes...
Circle the ones that apply:

Meditation	Yoga	Valuable Work	Seva	Exercise
Plant Food	Conscious Community		Regular Sleep	Laughter

How can you increase your personal dharma?

The difference between a resonant dharmic life and one subject to karmic influence is very clear. It is observed in your experience of vitality or lack. When a flower blooms, it grows and grows. It receives the sun and glorifies in its beauty for as long as the light is available. One miraculous aspect of dharmic living, is that light and warmth are available to you at all times. As we discussed prior, it takes discipline to see that this is the case. In the opposite set of conditions where karma is unregulated, you experience the world in terms of polarities.

The dharmic approach changes your relationship to time and space. Because you see beyond the trappings of polarities and are open to new possibilities, your energy is infused with effervescence. You may find yourself in perpetual motion. With practice and awareness you can observe the many cues from your subtle energy. With this increased sensitivity, you must re-learn how to care for your body-temple, the vessel through which you are able to experience your consciousness. You create a personal "road" which is aligned with the universal law of Dharma to manifest your intention.

SHUNIA & SAIBHANG
The fourth essential for the self - sensory being

Where we initiate from the practice of self-assessment

The Self-sensory human being consciously seeks to balance the great outward advances of the technological age with an equally strong connection to our inner human-ness. As the pressures of our outer environment increase—with ever-faster computers, more social networking opportunities, and instant global world news—an intentional, personal practice offers a powerful way to connect us back into our essential, multi faceted-self.

**The State of Shunia,
in the Words of Rumi:**

"You Are the Ocean in the Drop."

This path invites us to live a balanced life—not only between the inside and outside world, but in every way energy expresses itself. Our existence is a dance of complementary opposing forces called polarities. Within this dance of the polarities we navigate our transformation. Our reaction to the play is what causes our ease or disease, our expansion or our contraction. And this play is what we came here to master through balance. The balance point is the still point; shunia and it is not "reached" when one polarity overcomes the other. There is no winning or losing in this. Instead, the balance point is a state you drop into. The way to get there is completely unique to everyone and requires Self-reflection. There is no cookie-cutter way of transformation and there are no set rules to follow. What we suggest is that you create a deep awareness of your opportunities, transform the dis-harmonics, and dedicate, dedicate, and re-dedicate your time and energy to manifest your greatest, most balanced expression.

The yogic view is that the positive, negative and neutral (shunia) minds each have their way of expressing. This does not mean that the negative mind is bad and the positive mind is good, rather it means that they give you different information. We like to think of the positive mind as the projective mind and the negative mind as the protective mind. Your sensations are your guideposts along this journey to Purest Potential. It's important to be in right relationship with your feelings. Feelings are expressions of the mental process. When you can observe the expressions of your negative, positive and neutral minds then you can observe where your awareness is. This awareness allows you to create a devoted discipline that will consciously lead toward a regular, repeatable experience of shunia.

A Self-sensory being would read the signals in this way:

Energy Body	Negative Expression	Positive Expression	Neutral - Shunia
1	Dull	Smart	Creative
2	Disobedient	Obedient	Connected to Self
3	Don't use will	Use will	Bliss
4	Reactive	Conscious Action	Resurrection
5	Selfish	Martyr	Balance
6	Spaced out	Focused	Intuitive
7	Insecure	Secure	Self contained
8	Anxious	Energized	Courageous
9	Restless	Calm	Mastery
10	Shy	Determined	Radiant
11	Overwhelmed	Uplifting	Infinite

When you can observe your energy, you will *"know where you are at"*, and self initiate a practice, which allows you to dwell in Shunia. This will generate a new reference point, a new memory of expression for that energy body. Remember, there are two polarities- negative and positive and we are all unique expressions in how we dance these polarities.

A clear intention, combined with a daily yogic practice, and with pratyahar, requires Self-reflection and Self-initiation to stay the course.

> *Your devotion is the portal to enter Shunia, the essence of the experience of life.*

PRACTICE
From Polarity to Shunia

Write your answer to this question:

_____ (person's name) triggers me

to feel _____

Sit in easy pose with eyes $1/10^{th}$ open. Focus on tip of the nose.

Silently chant Wahe Guru in this way:

- On "Wa" mentally focus on the right eye.
- On "He" mentally focus on the left eye.
- On "Guru" mentally focus on the tip of the nose

10 Steps to Shunia

1) Inhale, exhale and mentally repeat Wahe Guru as described above.

2) Inhale and bring to mind the event which caused you to feel triggered.

3) Exhale and mentally repeat Wahe Guru as decribed above.

4) Inhale. Visualize and experience the actual feeling of the event.

5) Exhale and mentally repeat Wahe Guru as described above.

6) Inhale and reverse roles of the breakdown. Become the other person and experience their perspective.

7) Exhale and mentally repeat Wahe Guru as described above.

8) Inhale. Forgive the other person and forgive yourself.

9) Exhale and mentally repeat Wahe Guru.

10) Inhale. Let go of the incident and release it into the Universe.

The next step to create a breakthrough is to engage your energy from a state of shunia. First accept what is and then take action from a state of shunia, from peace.

1) Know what you don't want
2) Identify what you do want
3) Create a state of Shunia
4) Engage your energy as if it were already so
5) Be at peace and then take action

SAIBHUNG, "Self-initiation"

From shunia, we can observe where the opportunities for transformation are which can lead us to the final 'essential' - self-initiation.

In kundalini yoga no student is ever initiated; instead, we are encouraged to self-initiate. There are many reasons why this point about self-initiation is so important to a kundalini yogi. There is no teacher, book, friend, nor family that can make the ultimate difference in your life. At the moment of death—and each and every moment in life—it is you and you alone who can illuminate your experience and initiate yourself into *"I am, I am"*. When you affirm, *"I am, I am"* then you are relating from the light of your soul.

The attitude of self-initiation encourages your full participation in the enlightenment process because it requires a strong foundation to hold the increased frequency and magnetic power generated by the rising of the kundalini. 'With great power, comes great responsibility'. Your ability to respond in an enlightened way depends on the foundation upon which you stand.

Self-Initiate a strong foundation with these yogic essentials:

Intention, Pratyahar, Dharma and Karma, Shunia and Saibhang

1) **My intention is:**

2) My lifestyle is informed by pratyahar. **Five habits that rise me above the endless play of polarities:**

3) My dharma flows from my intention and allows me to travel with bright headlights - **My dharma is to:**

4) I understand what my karmic lessons are and don't take things personally - **My karmic lessons are:**

5) I have a daily practice to drop into Shunia where I observe my polarized reactions and recalibrate to neutral. **My daily practice is:**

6) I self-initiate and am the co-creator of my life. Yes! **My latest self-initiation is:**

With this foundation in place, you will be able to say, "Pass the popcorn" as you observe the movie of your life, instead of vanishing into the crazy drama of it all.

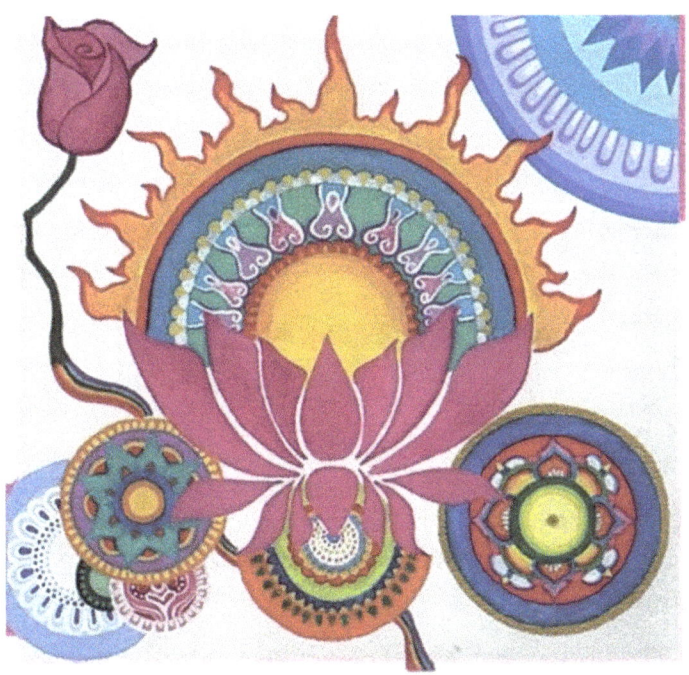

PRACTICE
Meditation to Balance Your Projection with Your Intention

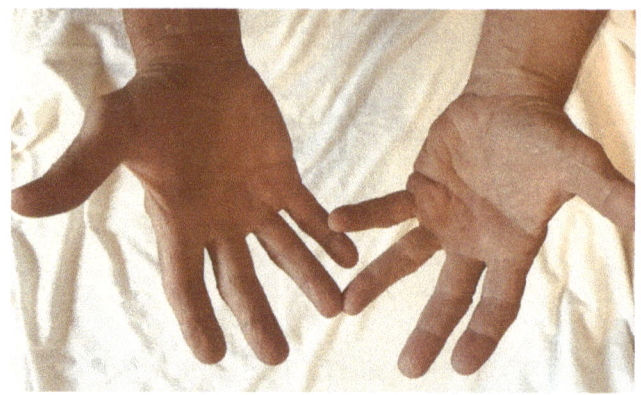

Sit in easy pose and bring the elbows relaxed at your sides, palms are flat and face up with the fingers spread gently.

Touch the tips of the ring fingers together with the right pinky under the left pinky not touching.

Close the eyes.

Chant 'SA, TA, NA, MA' in this way:

- On Sa tense the tip of the thumb and the index (Jupiter) finger,
- On Ta tense the tip of the thumb and the middle (Saturn) finger,
- On Na tense the tip of the thumb and the ring (Sun) finger,
- On Ma tense the tip of the thumb and the pinky (Mercury) finger.

Continue with this meditation for **3 to 11 minutes**.

Good Going!

With these four essentials:

1. Intention
2. Pratyahar
3. Dharma and Karma
4. Shunia and Saibhang

You have laid the groundwork to be your brilliant Self!

Take some time quiet time alone to rest,
meditate and integrate.

CHAPTER 3
ENGAGE THE ENERGY

The soul is constant and doesn't progress spiritually.
What can transform is all the 10 bodies when connected with the
light of the soul.

Our subtle anatomy illustrates that the human form has been designed with very specific ways to engage energy. Our energetic makeup consists of a vast spectrum of vibratory frequencies that constitute our wholeness—our complete vibratory signature. This spectrum is similar to the way a musical note is made up of not just one, but many frequencies vibrating together. Some frequencies are a higher vibration and some are lower. The fun begins when you realize how to contribute to this creative process by consciously engaging with your subtle anatomy—specifically the Chakras, Ten Bodies, and Nadis.

YOGIC ANATOMY OVERVIEW
The interaction of varying energies goes on all the time, everywhere in the body. The interchange, easily observed at the chakra points, is a sense of turning like a whirlpool in the middle of the sea. To get a better understanding of how to engage effectively with this subtle energy, it will help to have a wider view of yogic philosophy to understand the macrocosm and how the subtle anatomy operates. From this, it will become clear that there is a profound intention to the human design.

The 5 tattvas, 3 gunas, 7 chakras and 10 bodies all interact
automatically in harmony

The physical body needs food for it's sustenance
The soul needs prana for it's expression

Chakra System Analysis

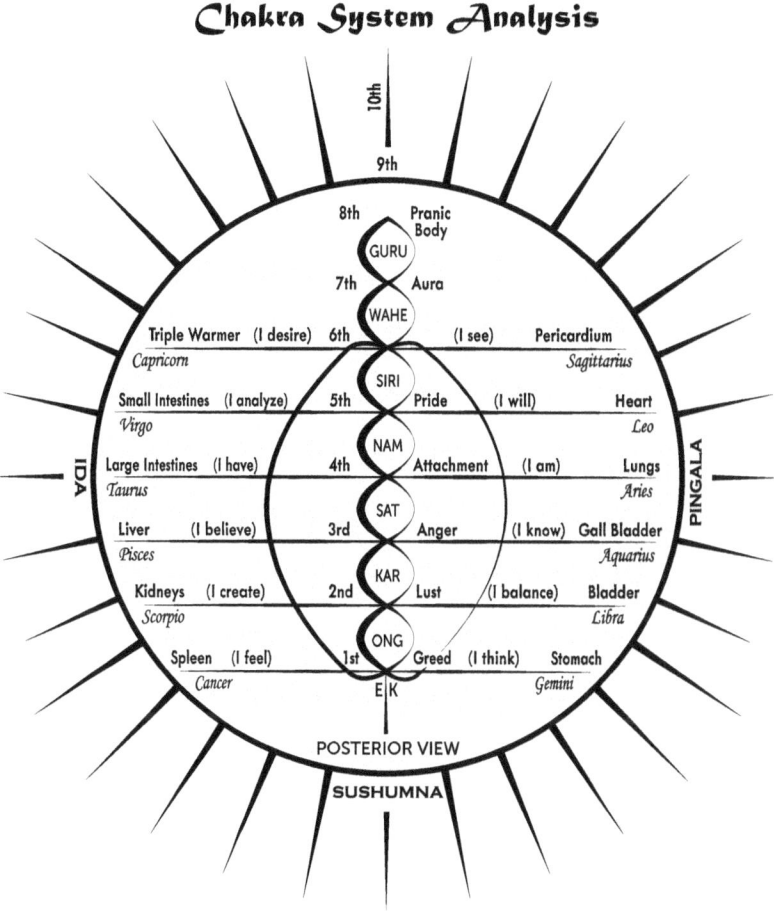

Yogic philosophy considers that prana is the soul, in fact, we are alive because of prana. It is through our Pranic Body that we 'ingest' universal prana into our being. From the Pranic Body it flows into the chakras, then prana flows out along the nadis, to energize the nervous system, the glandular system and the blood.

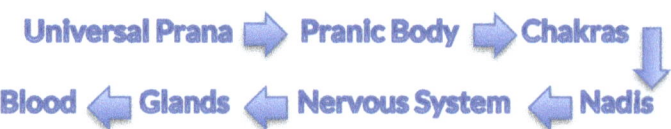

This energy flow chart clarifies the central importance of the Pranic Body, the chakras and nadis, as the distributors for prana from the subtle into the physical. With the self-sensory model in mind, awareness of this flow of energy becomes necessary. When exploring how to engage the energy, the most direct route is to discern the awareness each chakra provides. There are biological and emotional (and thus perceptual) consequences to the harmonic well being of each.

The chakras have a fixed location and a composite energetic make up. Each chakra is composed from the electric flow of two organs via meridian nodes, as well as those of the nerves and the local parts.

1st Chakra	Spleen meridian	Stomach meridian
2nd Chakra	Kidney meridian	Bladder meridian
3rd Chakra	Liver meridian	Gallbladder meridian
4th Chakra	Large Intestine Meridian	Lung meridian
5th Chakra	Small Intestine meridian	Heart meridian
6th Chakra	Triple Warmer meridian	Pericardium meridian

With healthy and balanced chakras, the energy that emerges is a byproduct of the health and balance of the constituent parts.

With the Ten Bodies, the energy itself is primary. They are embodied as an energetic force, complete with its own magnetic field. This is why we refer to them as "bodies." By recognizing these aspects of your psyche exist, and by opening a space for them in the physical world where they are more easily discussed and understood we can further enhance our experience as Self Sensory Beings.

BODY	LOCATION / EXPRESSION
1ST SOUL	1ST CHAKRA
2ND NEGATIVE MIND	2ND CHAKRA
3RD POSITIVE MIND	3RD CHAKRA
4TH NEUTRAL MIND	4TH CHAKRA
5TH PHYSICAL BODY	5TH CHAKRA
6TH ARC LINE	6TH CHAKRA
7TH AURA	AURA – GENERATED FROM THE CROWN
8TH PRANIC BODY AKA MAGNETIC FIELD	INFINITY FIGURE EIGHT WHICH INTERSECTS AT DIAPHRAGM
9TH SUBTLE BODY	SILVER OUTER LAYER OF AURA
10TH RADIANT BODY AKA CIRCUMVENT FORCE	GOLDEN RAYS WHICH EMANATE FROM OUTER EDGE OF AURA
11TH EMBODIMENT	COMMAND SPACE FOR ALL 10 BODIES TO BECOME INFINITE WITHIN YOURSELF

CHAKRAS AND THEIR EMANATIONS (BODIES)

When most books or teachers talk about chakras, they use symbolic language. "Chakra" literally means round, circle, or wheel. Ancient texts identify chakras as unseen wheels of energy located at precise points along a subtle energy channel that flows up and down through the spinal column. These wheels are the gears that operate the subtle machinery of yogic anatomy. They provide the link between the gross (physical) world and the subtler realms. The chakras are the location of conflict or harmony between interior reality and everyday life. There are many moving parts to the picture and each part creates its own electric pulse, which in turn, generates a magnetic field at each chakra. We call these magnetic fields the 'bodies'.

These complex structures consist of many constituent parts, both gross and subtle. It is important not to let the distinction between the touchable, bodily reality of meridians and organs become separated from the subtle, conceptual reality of the energetic forces.

Each chakra is comprised of opposing energetic frequencies in the meridians that come together. Energy from one electric circuit (meridian) spins clockwise at a chakra point where it meets with another electric circuit (meridian), spinning counterclockwise. This flow of electricity creates an electro-magnetic field that protects the flow of a Body. The actual physical organs associated with each of the meridians will reflect the balance or imbalance of the subtle anatomy established as a pattern of ease or dis-ease.

Knowing that your subtle anatomy is made up of the interplay of polarities, you can focus the power of your intention to neutralize your reaction to these polarities and navigate your dharmic path through this world of possibilities. The ancients observed that specific, intentional application of sound, breath, asana, and mudras created harmony while other sounds and activities created dis-harmony. By doing a yogic practice, you affect your subtle bodies to harmonize the spin of opposing electrical circuits.

FIRST CHAKRA

The usual story about Muldhara, or the Root Chakra, is its association with the individual's sense of security and well-being. Located just above the anal sphincter at the perineum, this chakra is where the stomach, spleen and pancreas meridians interact electrically. Considering these locations and parts, it is easy to see why this chakra is associated with feelings of security. The stomach is the governing member of the digestive system. The spleen and pancreas participate in the digestive process and also unite the digestive system with the glandular and immune systems, the systems that protect and maintain the body.

When everything functions as it should, the chakra and the energetics create the ability to eliminate that which is not needed. If this is not the case, then the location tells the story of the chakra's imbalance through physical, emotional and spiritual constipation. Literally and figuratively things close up.

Feeling insecure means security goes on high alert and often overreacts by perceiving threats when there may be none or standing down when a real threat appears. Insecurity means inflexibility—jumping to conclusions and an inability to switch gears when new information brings the truth of the matter to the surface. Basically, it means elimination becomes irregular as the body attempts to subconsciously hold onto or be rid of the matter at hand. Balancing the stomach and spleen/ pancreas meridians brings regularity and absolute security. Regularity is the self-discipline of the body and provides the confidence that any circumstance can be digested and the imbalances removed. A strong root chakra means the flexibility to embrace whatever happens.

~Soul Body - the emanation from the Root Chakra~

When you create balance, shunia, at the first chakra, your soul body can "speak" to you and become your best friend. It will be your touchstone for being human. Once you learn to identify the first body's energy within your being and listen to that inner guidance, you live in a state of harmony and happiness.

SECOND CHAKRA

The Swadisthana, or second chakra, is all about water and emotion. The analogy between water and emotion is a traditional one, and here it becomes quite literal. The second chakra is located two or three finger-widths below the navel and links the bladder and kidney meridian channels that tie into the sexual organs directly.

There is a sense of flow at work in the second chakra. The bladder regulates the movement of water and the kidneys manage the contents of that water. In terms of the emotion the second chakra will come into balance when fear is addressed. Because water symbolizes emotion itself, not a particular emotion, the ease and grace of flow can only be interrupted by what might make someone stand in the way of their own feelings. Of course this happens all the time. There is a big difference between emotional intelligence, which redirects that flow like the moon does the tides, and fear-based thinking and behavior, which swirls and agitates the flow like a storm over the ocean.

Location again shows the means of understanding why this chakra should operate this way. Being that this chakra is near to the organs of procreation, it makes sense that the relation to fear and emotion should arise. The need for people to love, connect, speak creatively, to be heard and to intercourse with each other is primal. And this goes deeper. Think of the way human cultures have understood the continuation of a family line. The necessity to carry on a family's lineage automatically places an undue burden and responsibility on an otherwise free life. The sense of need and struggle for survival, provides the first glimpse of fear from where other emotions will follow.

When the second chakra is balanced, the electricity from the nodes at the end of the bladder and kidney meridians churn this emotional energy. When we learn to channel our emotion into devotion then, our soul's journey becomes fearless and creates the deep connection to our true identity.

The Three Minds

The next three bodies are what ancient Indian texts refer to as the "threefold" or "three natures" of the mind. The process of navigating the 3 aspects of the mind are what Rishi Patanjali refers to as Samyama. The movement for a thought is that it passes through the negative, positive and then neutral aspects of the mind.

Like the kidneys, each mind performs a function. Also much like the Soul Body, each of these minds has a very specific energy. Seeing each associated with a chakra helps explain the respective roles of these minds as functioning mental capacities and as energetic projections of the self.

~Negative Mind – the emanation from the second Chakra~

As discussed above, the 2nd Body represents emotion as well as having its own particular emotional characteristics. Underlying the balance of energies at the 2nd Body is the question of what we call "longing to belong." This desire has a distinct origin in Indian philosophy. It is said to be the soul's misapprehension of itself as something other than God. In some circles, this is referred to as the "shadow."

Because the energetic balance at this Body affects one's general outlook and core emotional state, the volatility of an imbalanced 2nd Body has the potential to lead to a negative attitude, thus it's association with the Negative Mind. Energetic imbalance at this chakra evokes terms like "shadow," and is attributed to misperception. But it does not explain the function of that mind or the essential nature of that shadow energy.

The feeling of disconnection and sometimes a quick reactiveness arises when the 2nd Body is imbalanced. The Negative Mind, the 2nd Body, moves very quickly to assess the circumstances life provides. This is not an emotional response; it is only the act of analysis. If someone is reactive it is because the analysis has been hard wired to calculate danger in life. In the course of human

46

development, way back when, our primary concerns were survival, procreation, and protection of the family unit—the negative mind was the first aspect of the mind that developed.

A negative response to an emotion is potentially a natural response, but the function of the Negative Mind is as a safety mechanism—it is there merely to provide information so potential dangers can be assessed as quickly as possible. Functionally, it is easy to see that this mind is necessary and helpful. However, as an energetic body, the value of "negativity" is a little less clear.

The yogic way to process a thought is that it is essential for every thought to run its full course. Each thought arises and then passes through all three aspects of the mind —Negative Mind (2nd Body), Positive Mind (3rd Body) and Neutral Mind (4th Body). That means as a Body, the Negative Mind's job is to gather information. It has no decisions to make. Those decisions are best left to the Neutral Mind. Before the Neutral Mind makes a decision there is a weighing of the dangers, the role of the Negative Mind. The balanced expression of the Negative Mind creates the deepest connection to the light of our soul.

THIRD CHAKRA

The Manipura, traditionally called the Nabhi and known as the third chakra, is located at the navel and is the focal point of a host of nerves that surround the solar plexus. Besides the organs that link up at this chakra, these nerves provide a great deal of awareness. This is why it is commonly said, "he went with his gut." The traditional view of the third chakra is that it is the center of a person's sense of power and authority, just as the second and first chakras were linked by the behaviors exhibited, the third chakra when in or out of balance manifests as either confidence and precise energetic projection or a lack thereof.

The location of this chakra is clearly emblematic of the relationship between the physical and the not physical. The third chakra puts a capstone on what is referred to as "the lower triangle", made up of the lower three chakras.

The gall bladder interacts electrically in the third chakra and is a pretty innocuous organ, in the eyes of Western medicine. Many people have it removed and continue to live long lives without its aid. The gall bladder's simple function is to store the liver's bile and help break down complex materials like fats before they reach the liver. It is like the apprentice to the master artist. The apprentice, the gall bladder, carves the stone into form so the master can add the finishing touches, the skilled touches only a master has. The liver is the other organ that interacts electrically in the third chakra. Perhaps the most complicated organ in the body, after the brain, the liver is charged with many jobs to perform: to absorb proteins, detoxify the blood, and help regulate metabolism. These are just a few of the liver's digestive, glandular and hemodynamic responsibilities. The picture painted here is of the liver being the powerhouse and another, the gall bladder, whose specific job it is to support the powerhouse. This story is very telling when relating to third chakra.

Power is potential energy. The human body cannot survive without a functioning liver, which makes it clear that this organ provides a certain amount of potential to the whole human system by itself. The gall bladder has the job to make the liver more efficient and to make the potential more potent.

This picture of a relationship is fitting for describing the ways in which a balanced electrical current in the third chakra makes itself known. Not so long ago when someone was particularly nasty, people would say they had a lot of bile. This substance within the gall bladder helps the liver perform its many tasks. Bile can seep into the liver and make digestion sometimes a painful experience. The implication of an imbalanced third chakra is similar to a digestive state of intolerance. Whatever the situation is, it doesn't want to go down. This can create anger or a sense of being forsaken. When the third chakra is balanced, ease pervades. Acceptance brings friendliness.

48

~Positive Mind - the emanation from the third Chakra~

As the energetic 3rd Body, the Positive Mind, provides morale and an uplifting assessment of the potential in any given situation. Like the gung-ho athlete who believes the team can accomplish any task. The Positive Mind takes success as a given and looks past any difficulties to a successful outcome. It is a perfect compliment to the Negative Mind, whose great concern is self-protection and what might go wrong.

This is not to say that the Positive Mind has no drawbacks. There is an excessively optimistic, "greener grass" mentality dominating here. If this energetic body just projects positivity in all directions, two things will happen. First, the person attached to this positive mind will run out of energy trying to make every projection a reality. Second, in the face of a disappointment, the emotion that has become attached to the outcome will transfer its negative energy to that which has been ignored, the Negative Mind, and often result in self-critique.

The emotions attending the balance of the 3rd Body are based on relationship to others. The projection from the emotional influence of the Positive Mind entails either a desire to please others or to see the self in a certain relationship with others. When attached to a particular projection that person becomes rigid, intolerant of others' views and opinions, and can even get angry when advice is offered. The Positive Mind needs the devotion of the 4th Body, just like the Negative Mind does. The Positive Mind's projection is powerful and needs to be balanced with deep acceptance of the circumstances in a given situation. A determination to perceive things realistically can be developed a number of ways. Here at the 3rd Body, our psyche helps refine the ability to interpret that gut feeling and check the Positive Mind's projection.

As an energetic body, the Positive Mind provides morale and an uplifting assessment of the potential in a given situation. The potential we speak of here is the experience of bliss, not just happiness.

49

FOURTH CHAKRA

The Anahata, or Heart Chakra, is the balance point for the whole chakra system. Just as the first, second and third chakras make up the "lower triangle," there is a "higher triangle" composed of the topmost chakras. Generally speaking, the higher the chakra, the subtler the energy Body is. This is evident in the kinds of emotions that tag along with the balance in each Body. Here at the heart, there is another balancing act taking place—one that suggests the energies of the upper and lower chakras must be aligned for the Anahata to be in energetic harmony.

The organs whose meridians have an electric relationship to the heart chakra are the lungs and large intestine. These meridians generate the relationship between the upper and lower chakras and the subtle element of air and the less subtle elements of earth, water and fire. The interaction with the elements is suggestive to these organs' bodily functions. The lungs obviously supply the means by which life can take place. The energy drawn from the air is like the fuel taken from the food broken down in its final stages by the large intestine. So if the large intestine's function is to squeeze the last little bit of relevant energy from food and leave behind only matter to be eliminated from the body, the question becomes: Is this similar to the breathing process and the functions of the psyche that each organ embodies?

It is easy to imagine the lungs themselves performing this function. However, the connotation here is that the process is finely tuned with an acute focus on its relative efficiency. This is a major reason why conscious breathing is such an integral part of yoga practice. By attuning the lungs to an efficient practice, the fourth chakra becomes more balanced which influences the balance of the whole chakra system.

By balancing this chakra there is an ease of mind that signifies equilibrium throughout the system. From the bottom-up there is a sense of steadiness anchored in the removal of all that does not serve the body. When the 4th Chakra is out of balance, or the lungs and large intestine meridians are not working properly, the effect is a relatively unsteady mental outlook. From the opposite perspective, what the 4th Chakra promises is a deep compassion defined as a life "with passion".

The sense of compassion influences the balance of the 4th Chakra. The organs' focus on efficient absorption of energy is what this Chakra provides—its whole foundation, the entire means of confident energetic projection, stems from efficient absorption of prana.

~Neutral Mind - the emanation from the fourth Chakra~

When both the Negative and Positive Minds are in balance they simply relate a series of facts—the drawbacks and benefits of a situation or choice. For example, when buying a car the Negative Mind is very important because it weighs the costs, the character of the salesman, and the evident durability of the vehicle. The negative mind can be turned on for the buyer to balance any over-eagerness with the purchase. On the other hand, the Positive Mind sees the bright paint job, the powerful motor, and how being seen in this car would improve your reputation. It sees that fun and excitement on the open road, absent any emotion, is pretty cool. This is where the Neutral Mind comes in handy. It says, "hey, I deserve to enjoy the open road, but the insurance it takes to cover a sports car costs a lot more than the other options." The Neutral Mind weighs the need for space and economy against the option of a two-door hatchback with poor gas mileage. The Neutral Mind notices that there is a four-door hybrid on the other end of the lot that has additional safety features, better insurance rates, gets great mileage, and aligns with your higher ideals! Having allowed the negatives to come up, and calmly taken note of the positives, you can approach the decision-making process with more clarity and even discover new solutions.

The 4th Body is an effective decision maker, because it requires absolute honesty. As the Negative and Positive Mind come into balance—both within themselves and with each other—much of the work has been done, but not quite done yet. If only two opposing bodies were available than there would be a constant, tumultuous, and energetic back and forth. That is why it is important to cultivate an experience of the Neutral Mind. The more in touch with its presence you become, the easier it is to recognize the charge of emotion that comes along with any individual thought. The Neutral Mind is like an abacus—it can only add and subtract the data given to it by the Negative and Positive Minds. In neutrality, the heart weighs in and the right decision often just presents itself. By fostering the experience of a Neutral Mind in life, the drama of a coworker and the flirtatious relationship at the coffee shop disappears. In each moment you'll have the option to not participate in these mini-dramas. Instead, when you do choose to engage, you can bring compassionate energy into the situation.

As previously mentioned, the quality of compassion is the balance point for the heart's attendant emotions. By cultivating a devotional Neutral Mind, which allows the Positive and Negative Minds to present information with no judgment, understanding unfolds. Steady patience dominates while the facts are coming in. When dealing with deadlines and everyday life, a practiced Neutral Mind allows an understanding through the heart and because this rhythmically occurs, there is an appreciation for harmony—the gift within the circumstances. You then live as a yogi, unaffected by the polarities of life.

FIFTH CHAKRA

> Meditation removes the barrier between the known and the unknown and gives you intuitive infinity.

The fifth chakra is the touch point for the heart and small intestine meridians. Curiously, the heart chakra does not link up to the heart by the way of meridians. Instead, the heart finds itself connected along with the small intestine to the Vishuddha, or Throat Chakra. The logic of this lies in the subtlety of the ascending chakras' energies.

The throat is a passage for air and food. As with the other Bodies and chakras, there is a relationship between gross matter and unseen forces at work here. It is important to note that the throat is a two-way street and the human voice is the primary energy that flows through the throat.

As described earlier, the large intestine's function is the last stage for the absorption of energy and the place where useful energy is absolutely separated from the superfluous. The small intestine is where the majority of this energetic absorption takes place. The heart is the rhythm-maker for life. When someone is genuine his or her actions are "heartfelt." There is an essence formed of these organs, both from matter into energy and from experience into spirit. In other words, the heart is not just the physiological organ but also the experiential essence of having a heart itself. The lungs have their role to play in the absorption of energy from the air; the throat has a similarly transformative role, as it passes the air to and from the lungs. With the process of deeply digesting, not just the physical sense but in extracting an essence, the small intestine and heart disperse as the identity that is perceptible in the body. Likewise with words, the embodiment of identifying can only reach fruition through the voice. Words codify an experience and when the 5th Chakra is in balance, the use of language is precise and effective.

~Physical Body - the emanation from the fifth Chakra~

What has been presented is a provocative picture: a soul outfitted with three minds before it even receives a body. There is an implied space between the soul and the physical body, made up of the mind. There are gradations between body and soul that like the chakras, move upward with increasing subtlety. Given this observation and the western tendency to differentiate body and soul, the placement of the Physical Body may seem strange. However, looking past the western dynamic "split" and recalling the Ten Bodies as individuated energies, it is plain to see that the physical body is merely a shell built to house the soul and mind. Like the other Bodies in the Ten Bodies system, the physical body is a force and one that is able to literally touch others, pick things up, move them around, or to drive an ecological hybrid car.

Given that the physical body literally does things, the emotions attendant to the 5th Body are especially telling. The outlook supplying these emotions hinges on action. The energy in the physical body is either advancing in clarity and upliftment or retreating in critical timidity. Generally speaking, thoughts and feelings emerge and the principal way the mind has of understanding these thoughts and feelings is through language. It is then through connection with the energetic physical body—the 5th Body—that it is possible, in word and deed, for truth and intention to be made manifest on the physical plane.

The implications for this are astounding and literally reverberating. The 5th Body and the physical body and the human larynx—the voice-box—all have a role in creating the quality of truth through actual, physical vibration. The media for truth are perceptible in different ways, each requiring refinement of the senses. The picture all this provides is of a body, a physical body, which is an energetic vessel for truth. It is the power of embodiment, of symbol, and it is a power that can be developed—both in actual physical form and through words.

We now know that our psyche has a soul, three minds, and a physical body that contains them. According to Yogic understanding the first five chakras and the resulting Bodies must be balanced energetically on a daily basis in order to neutralize our reactive patterns to the events of life. Once this balance is achieved, the 6th body, the arc line opens access to cosmic knowledge and will start to oversee the first five Bodies. This, in turn, allows for your excellence and abundance with each and every breath.

SIXTH CHAKRA

The refinement of the chakras continues as the sixth chakra—the Ajna chakra or "Third Eye"—comes into view. The sixth chakra is located precisely at the site of the pituitary gland. Instead of connecting to a particular organ, the meridians tie this "seat of wisdom" to the entirety of the glandular and nervous systems. This chakra at its functional level links the regulatory functions of the body to its sense of self, its awareness.

There are many parts to be considered when describing the total energy of the 6th Body's magnetic field. The pituitary, also known as the "master gland", has an incredibly powerful and very complex set of functions. We know that the nervous and glandular systems meet by way of the meridians. This relationship describes how the sympathetic and parasympathetic nervous systems interact. Their electric signals—both voluntary and involuntary—communicate through the pituitary gland, maintaining relative stasis in the whole body. The profound role of this "seat of awareness" is partially due to the volume of information it processes and precisely its relative ability to achieve balance.

The sixth Chakra is named agiaa chakra. Agiaa means: to sanction. Life will be protected when it is projected from a connection to the third eye.

The meridians tie the sixth chakra to the glandular system via the San Jiao, or Triple Warmer, so called because it is divided into three parts. Each of these subsequent parts is both an energy field and a set of glands grouped together according to the function each performs in aid of the internal organs for respiration, digestion, and elimination. The glands that make up these groupings act like any other glands: they secrete the right chemicals at the right time to assist organ protection, function, and upkeep. The other meridian present in the sixth chakra links directly to the pericardium, the pouch surrounding the heart and lungs. The primary role of the pericardium is the protection of the heart and the lungs by surrounding it with a pouch of protective fluid that assists in ease of function and lubrication. By virtue of its location, the pericardium is also inextricably connected to the phrenic nerves, which link directly to the brain.

Since the 6th Chakra has so much information passing through it, it is no wonder that intuition is considered a cardinal virtue. It also makes sense that the pituitary is considered the "master gland." In fact, the Triple Warmer unites the vital organs in a single system and the pericardium ties the essence of life, the breath of life via cardio-pulmonary function, to the function of awareness, the brain and nervous system. The 6th Chakra has a particular kind of power—it protects and projects – it brings us all we need through its power to attract and then manifest our thoughts into our reality.

The way that this whole Body is constructed is practically insistent that the pituitary, the master gland of the body, be just that—a master.

The connection between glandular function and the nervous system is absolute. The emotions are attendant to the relative balance of each system and the whole Body. When the nervous system is out of balance it becomes erratic, resulting in nervousness and anxiety, as opposed to a calm, cool, and collected disposition. Similarly, an imbalanced glandular system can make a person commotional, which makes sense given the regular function of the glandular system. The triggered commotion can release hormones and other neuro-chemicals that secrete and undermine overall health. If the experience of emotion is commotion caused by Chakra imbalances, the results are not fun. However, positive emotions such as devoted emotional energy to your own excellence can be cultivated and these results are not only fun, but also full of bliss.

We learn through disciplined living—directing emotion to devotion—to command fulfilling results from the events of life. Energetically speaking, this means unifying all the body's functions into a single frequency. So the awareness promised by the third eye gives each person not only a way to observe and maintain the body's functions, but also supplies the answers about how to realize enlightenment. We realize enlightenment through self-illumination or commanding the psyche in its interface with life to experience bliss from the events it faces.

~Arc Line - the emanation from the sixth Chakra~

The arc line was perceived as a halo by ancient sources in the western tradition. The arc line is a thin band of intensely concentrated electromagnetic energy created by 9 to 11 rays of light that project out of the third eye. This band crosses the forehead from ear to ear in the shape of an arc. This band is only millimeters wide but contains a concentrated, energetic link to all the rest of the Ten Bodies. In other words, it functions within the Ten Bodies system in a manner that provides a place where the totality links up, at the edge of the gross and the subtle. In this arc line both realms can be reached and maximum awareness becomes possible.

As with the other Bodies, there is an emotional charge to the relative balance of the third eye. The systems are supplying this awareness already; it just takes practice to observe it all. This border territory is where the heavens can be perceived touching the earth, it is where the veil is thinnest.

Mastery of the pituitary and experiencing the energy of the arc line occurs through the access afforded by meditation. Meditation stimulates the optic nerve, which in turn activates the pituitary gland, creating focus, a seeing from the third eye. The vision this practice creates allows the practitioner's inner sight, the intuition, to awaken. The process can lead to an inner world of deep concentration or focus on what the light of our soul desires to manifest in this lifetime. Mastery of that interior realm unfolds, creating the ability to focus both on our spiritual as well as our worldly lives. Many of the kundalini meditation practices can balance the 6th Body and give the experience of deep focus to whatever endeavor we apply our self. Mastery of that interior realm unfolds, passing into the outer and allows for the processing of a vast amount of awareness. A deep meditation practice balances the Chakra and provides an experience of the Arcline, which can become viscerally present and is said to be the energetic embodiment of prayer.

THE SEVENTH CHAKRA

The activation of this chakra is directly associated with the ignition of the inner flame, also called "the light within." The Sahashara, or "crown" chakra, is associated with the pineal gland. This gland is situated between the brain's hemispheres, receiving light through a channel at the top of the skull. In mystical traditions, this pine-cone-shaped gland is linked intimately with human enlightenment. The exact functions in the body are not yet fully determined, except to say that it helps stabilize the body's inner clock and releases serotonin. The suggestion of the "thousand-petaled lotus" is that enlightened life is a constant unfolding, like the petals of a flower opening to greet the sun. There are no specific bodily meridians that tie into this chakra.

~Aura - the emanation from the seventh Chakra~

The rays projecting out from the crown chakra create the aura, which is said to electromagnetically protect not only the meridian functions of the 6 Chakras, but also the balance of the chakras. The aura creates a sense of containment, which is experienced from the electrical system. So, we use the word self-containment - since the self is the balance of the first five chakras and directed by the 6th Chakra. The chakra system is electric as it creates a voltage and the 7th body is electromagnetic. This is the field that protects the functionality of the voltage in the chakras.

THE SUBTLE BODIES, 8,9,10

As we explore the 8th Body, the Pranic Body; the 9th Body, the Subtle Body; and the 10th as the Radiant Body we see a very detailed, protective system for maintaining the delicate and sophisticated balance that can serve the brilliance of self – realization. The "voltage "of life is based upon the pranic body. The "mastery" of life is based on the 9th body and the light of the soul, when expressed through the radiant body, brings constant success.

The soul does not reside in just one part of the body. It is a huge volume of light that reflects in many different colors. At any one time it 'beams' at one part of the psyche, more powerfully than at any other part. The soul is named the 'beam center' of the spirit. If the 'beam center' is focused at the Ajna chakra, it will generate a strong intuitive sense. When the beam center is on the heart chakra it means that the person is very much in love, of service and generous. Non-meditators usually have multiple, weaker beams and an intentional meditation practice can generate that one beam aligned with our Purest Potential.

This is why a strong everyday yogic practice is so important. It provides the foundation that promotes healthy lifestyle habits, which ensure the proper functioning of each organ, which then creates a more powerful electric pulse at the end of each meridian/nadi. This then, demands that the energy of each chakra is balanced according to the increased power. A powerful aura provides more stability to the chakras. Turning up the power allows the spin of each vortex to be less like a whirlpool, and more like pair of turbines spinning side-by side in opposite directions. The result of this electric turbine motion is that it draws the Kundalini upward through the shushmuna nadi channel. When this vital frequency passes through the energy field of each chakra, it produces a side effect, what the ancient yogis called "ras" literally meaning, "juice" or "nectar." At this point, not only is each organ healthy and every passageway clear, the energy bodies get balanced and you can enjoy your whole Self—physically and energetically. The ancient texts describe the chakras as gates through which the life energy of the universe flows. In short, when you create a conscious lifestyle and care for the body, as well as balance the chakras and their energy Body emanations, you ensure an experience of your purest potential, your brilliance.

You become a beacon of light with
a well developed radiant body.

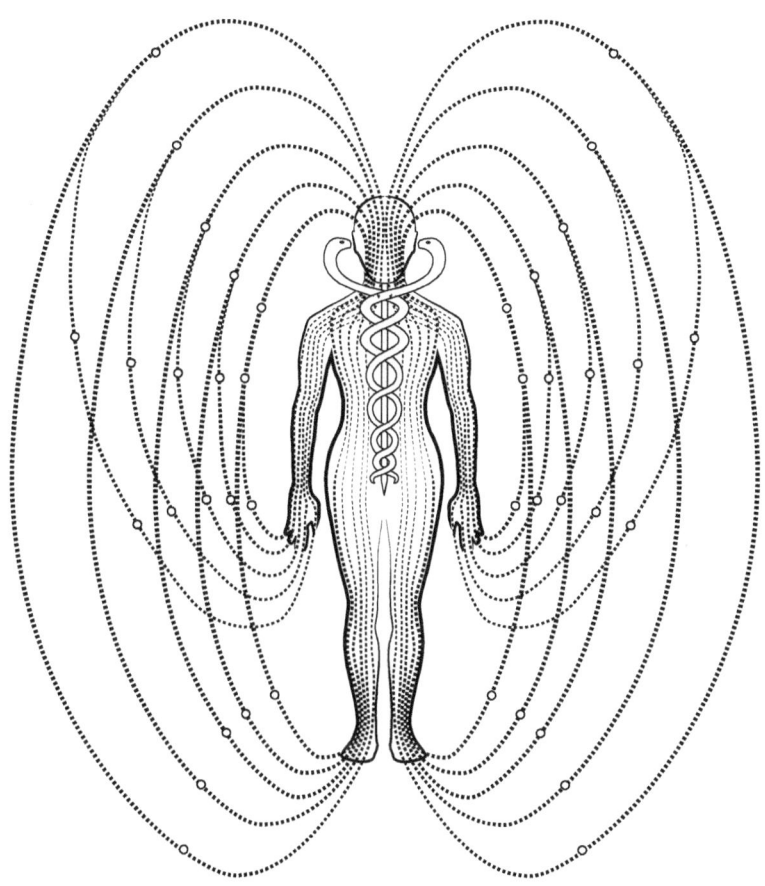

NADIS

After the prana whirls through the chakras, it disburses deeper into the body via the nadis. These nadis conduct energies of various types throughout the body. In Chinese medicine the nadis are called meridians and connect to the chakras, as illustrated in the previous chart.

In terms of yogic anatomy, the three primary nadis are described as a sacred Trinity: the ida, pingala, and shushmuna— relating to Brahma, Vishnu, and Shiva. The chakras are where the two subtle energy channels intersect with the central channel, respectively the ida, pingala and shushmana nadis. The Ida and Pingala nadis carry complimentary energies; Ida is cooling and soothing, Pingala is stimulating and energizing. When harmony between these two energies occurs at the chakra centers, we observe normal functioning of the organs and an increase in the size of the protective magnetic field (Body).

The movement of these two channels, the Ida and Pingala, intertwines like a series of figure eights that start at the base of the spine, moving from side to side and intersecting at each chakra. Each nadi tracks through the pineal and pituitary glands, with the left nadi ending at the left nostril and the right nadi at the right nostril. The ida and pingala govern all the other nadis and are responsible for left brain/right brain predominance. The left, or lunar nadi (ida) dominates right-brain activity, which is feeling-oriented. The right or solar nadi (pingala) dominates left-brain activity and is rationally oriented. Within the shushmuna nadi the kundalini rises provoked by the energetic polarities at the bottom-most point of each nadi.

In the western medical tradition, these nadis are represented by the caduceus. This symbol—carried by the messenger of god, from both the Greek and Roman traditions—can be viewed as a map, laying out very specifically the path of these channels. The image is that of a staff with two snakes coiled around it.

The best way to experience the subtle anatomy is by following the path of the breath. This structure can be more fully understood by your experience of it.

We will connect with the energy of the Ida nadi first. Block off the right nostril and breathe long and deep through the left nostril only. Observe.

Close off the left nostril and breathe long and deep through the right nostril only. Observe.

Another process comes into play where the Ida and pingala nadis cross at the chakras. Through pranayam, conscious breathing, the central channel or shushmuna can be activated. Imagine the shushmuna is your biggest electrical conductor. The fluid that protects this system is called the cerebral spinal fluid. It is the electrical force of the kundalini energy, which keeps the normal flow of this fluid moving properly to bathe the tissues and structures with necessary nutrients. With a practice of Kundalini yoga we enhance this flow by energetically harmonizing imbalances at the chakras.

SAMSKARAS- the wheel of time

There is another phenomena within the yoga world that is described as a wheel named "samskara." On the micro level, samskaras are the mental constructions that people develop, whether consciously or unconsciously, which express as karmic imbalances of the chakras. However, on the widest scale there is one samskara, the "wheel of time"; a symbol so pervasive in Indian culture that it appears on the national flag to this day. The importance of the dynamics of time cannot be underestimated here. Because you are a being made of flesh and blood, the materials of this earth, there is a part of you that is subject to time and space.

The passage of time has its effect on the physical body much like environmental conditions have an effect on a physical structure. It is easy to fall into the trap of routine living, where time is master. When that happens, life's subtleties are ignored which allows the physical body and corresponding chakras, as well as other gross and subtle systems, to fall into disharmony. When the bubble of protection, provided by the magnetic field from balanced chakras, dissolves, all that is left is matter—organs and blood and maybe a little space. If this happens, you become subject to the laws of time and space and there is more wear and tear on your body parts. Over time, the friction of imbalanced energy generates heat which creates inflammation and at the microscopic level, molecular breakdown.

Looking at samskaras on the microcosmic level, you can ignore the subtleties of life allowing the wheel of time to create wear and tear on your system, or you can choose to dedicate your focus to maintain your subtle anatomy and minimize unconscious disharmony. The inner wheels, the chakras, are not simple body mechanisms but complex structures consisting of many constituent parts, both gross and subtle. By engaging these subtle structures, especially with devotional commitment, one can achieve better health and a whole world of possible opportunities opens up to further self-awareness and personal development. Paths unfold to offer seemingly infinite means to Self initiate your brilliance; strategies will be discussed further for contextualizing this opportunity.

> *Life is connected to the soul when it's experienced with a well developed subtle body.*

PRACTICE
Engage your Energy

It is so easy to spend too much time fixated on what is wrong, on what is not working. All we have to do is check the news. Ask yourself: Is my awareness like the daily news focused on what I need to heal and fix? Examples: anger, depression, physical toxins?

Instead could you devote time in this way:
Spend 10% of your time to notice the disharmony and commit the other 90% to create your intentional life, the life you want.

What would have to change?

When you engage your energy intentionally it will bring your focus within, instead of trying to control the outside environments.

A Process for Transformation:
- Observe a past experience which causes disharmony
- Visualize a new more harmonic expression
- Commit to a specific yogic practice to harmonize the energy

The yoga practice needs to be done daily for at least 40 days to generate the psychic heat, what yogis call tapasia, needed to balance the imbalance at the chakra.

The main point is that each of the Chakras and Ten Bodies are readily available to experience. Engaging with these energies is a profound step in the healing process and can provide a foundation for moving forward towards a life of brilliance.

By breaking down the hard boundary between body, mind, and soul we have elucidated an enormous field of teachings for exploration and self-discovery. As you see and experience these new models for self-understanding, you can conduct experiments to explore this relationship to better develop the awareness of consciousness.

By recognizing the multiple layers of subtlety at work within these various human systems, it also becomes clear that there is a profound organization at work. With this map of the body's subtle energetic systems, it will be much more natural to take preventative measures to ensure health and keep the energy of each of the Ten Bodies, chakras, nadis and individual organs balanced. To take that experience and translate it into a lifestyle based on positive daily habits is the journey of a self-sensory human.

Chapter 4
TURN UP THE BRILLIANCE

The Thesaurus suggests these words for brilliance: beam, excellence, inspiration, intelligence, radiance, glow and wisdom. We suggest that you make brilliance into an intention. It is something to realize. This journey is not a sequential "leveling up" through the chakras to reach some special enlightenment place. Each chakra is vital to the proper functioning of all the other chakras; there is no higher or lower chakra, this system is a holistic integrated structure. What we suggest is that you have the intention to ignite Purest Potential, which then creates a constant awareness of how the polarities within and without are affecting you and that you develop the capacity to create shunia. This is a process. Each breath, each thought and each action presents an opportunity to find that still point, by unwinding the effects of this polarized duality. Living with the awareness that you can choose to dwell in light, is "brilliance."

The yogis compare the experience of shunia to a swan, the 'hans'. The swan remains dry while in the water—she is in the water but not affected or changed by it; just so we can be in the world, but not of it. Shunia is the experience of neutrality, which is expressed from the integration of polarities at each of the chakras. It is this neutrality, which facilitates the kundalini to rise.

Brilliance happens when you experience that you are light and when as a multi-faceted being, you magnify that light through the ten energy bodies. This is a process that unfolds in a series of 5 padas, or 5 stages:

Saram Pad	**Karam Pad**	**Shakti Pad**
	Sahej Pad	**Sat Pad**

Observe in the chart how this process to develop your radiance is similar to cultivating any relationship. First you experience the honeymoon phase, then there is the actual making it real phase, followed by the very critical power struggle, only then can there be true ease and balance and then final mastery. Each phase needs to be gone through and mastered and just a heads up: this process is never actually done. As long as you are alive there will be endless opportunities for deepening of these "padas".

Essence of Pada	Learning	Challenges	Qualities to Cultivate
Saram Pad Novice, feel "happy"	Called on to do, learn, explore Simple instructions, Set goals	What to focus on? Give priority to? Devotion is tested	Obedience to teachings Motivation
Karam Pad Apprentice, "doing". Practice the discipline	Interaction to process experiences, make time to practice	Learning new perceptions, karmas are tested. See where you need to grow	Discipline to do regular practice
Shakti Pad Practitioner, "doubt". Power struggle	Ability to choose a goal, fix on a motivation, commit to a set of values, develop humility	Test of power Overcoming attachments Overcoming doubt Spiritual ego, Testing ability to sacrifice	Commitment to higher values of teachings, journey navel to heart
Sahej Pad Expert "Grace/balance"	Commit to teach where you need to leap	To keep beginners mind	Intuition Compassion
Sat Pad Master "harmony"	Merging with Self, lead and serve a community	Test of Humility	Neutral mind

This process of 5 stages is a difficult concept in the West where we so often demand instant gratification. You may notice that many yoga centers offer versions of "instant gratification yoga." It takes no time on the Internet to find studios offering purely physical benefits. These physical benefits from yoga are experienced much more immediate and have a definite appeal to our fast-moving society.

Another challenge around this concept of brilliance or enlightenment is how to actually teach it. What we find is that especially the English language is limited in its ability to express any experience of the sacred. The Sanskrit language has ninety-six words for love; ancient Persian has eighty, Greek three, and English has only one. Language cannot easily convey what an experience of enlightenment is, so we follow what Patanjali Rishi figured out ages ago: the fewer words used the better. Our role is not to describe what enlightenment is, but to show you a way to do that, which yogis and mystics have done for ages—to fill in the blanks with your own experiences.

No one's journey to enlightenment can ever be the same; we each came into being for our own unique expression of our brilliance. So yes, the ultimate experience of yoga—enlightenment—is in the gradual awakening of your kundalini, the life force energy in self-realization. And self-realization expresses itself usually, as a unique process rather than an instantaneous event. It takes time to strengthen the nervous system so that it can handle the higher voltage of increased awareness. Let's review how the kundalini rises.

KUNDALINI

Kundalini yoga harmonizes and coordinates all of the ten bodies into the oneness of your life.

Kundalini means coiled energy; imagine that this Central Biorhythm is an unlimited coil that separates itself into smaller coils whose energy you can direct to experience infinity. If that coiled energy is joined with the seat of the soul, the pineal gland, the glandular system will combine with the nervous system to create such a sensitivity that the brain will receive signals and integrate them to a new and permanent level of awareness. It is the raising of the kundalini, which awakens the creative potential in a person.

A student in Santa Fe told us that she has a client who in the last six months had made more money then she ever imagined. This now-very-wealthy client in the same breath told her that she is still missing "it." She always thought that money would get her "it." Now she has all the money yet "it" is still missing from her life. What is it that drives us to experience more, and to keep looking for that which we can't even describe?

As yogis we call this force the kundalini, the spiritual nerve energy that resides within the subtle anatomy of each person. The kundalini energy ascends, turns on our brilliance, creates expansion and then descends and brings balance and new life to each chakra.

To raise the kundalini is not hard to do, some have fallen on their bottom, which caused it to rise, and others have done it by using mind-altering substances. These days more and more people are having spontaneous experiences of the kundalini rising. To have this energy rise all of the sudden can be very disruptive and sometimes damaging. The voltage of the kundalini is VERY increased from 'normal' consciousness. A regular practice of kundalini yoga prepares the nervous system to handle this increased voltage so that integration can occur. The way to live with this energy engaged and continue to expand; is what this book is about.

PRACTICE

The visualization will take you through the 3 granthis, which are the locations for the 3 psychic knots, which are the blockages on the path of the awakened kundalini. The granthis are named brahma, vishnu and shiva, and are located in the etheric body at the root chakra, the heart chakra and the third eye.

1) Brahma granthi functions in the region of muladhara, the 1st chakra. It implies feeling stuck and uncreative. The application of the mulabandha, root lock, helps to clear the blockages at the Brahma granthi.

2) Vishnu granthi operates in the region of anahata , the 4th chakra. It is associated with being caught in the polarities of life. The application of the Uddhiyana bandha, diaphragm lock, helps to clear the blockages at the Vishnu granthi.

3) Shiva granthi functions in the region of ajna, the 6th chakra. It is associated with a lack of focus and confusion. The application of Jullundur bandha, neck lock, helps to clear the blockages at the Shiva granthi.

There have been many descriptions of how the kundalini rises and what happens when it does. What follows is a composition of the kundalini teachings about this process. This is best experienced as a meditation with perhaps a friend reading the following while you breathe and visualize. You will need to know how to apply the 'bandhas' and can find that process explained in the appendix.

Take a few minutes to become very still and bring your focus on your breath.

Take several long deep breaths. Inhale wide and exhale tall.

Let the breath attune you to your subtle energy. Inhale wide, exhale tall.

Observe the spine, the inside and the outside. Breathe into the spine and observe the energy present. Inhale wide, exhale tall.

While sitting perfectly straight, inhale, hold the breath, and apply mulabandh, root lock.

Feel how this bandha draws Prana down from the heart area to the navel chakra, the pranic center, and the starting point for 72000 nadis. Observe the vitality of this pranic center, breathe into this experience for a few long deep breaths.

Relax the breath.

Now only apply mulabandh at the end of the exhalation. Hold the breath out and apply root lock. Observe how this bandhed breathing draws the apana up from the muladhara chakra to the third chakra.

Continue to apply mulabandh at the end of the exhale for a few more breaths and tune into the expression of apana.

Relax the breathing. Observe the energetic difference between prana and apana.

Begin to apply mulabandh at the top of the inhalation and at the end of the exhale.

Feel how this interaction of prana and apana, being opposing pranic forces, creates a tremendous heat in the third chakra. Continue for a few minutes until you experience this heat.

Note how this heat awakens the kundalini and starts her journey from the area of the navel chakra down to the root chakra. Pay attention to this movement, and continue this bandhed breath.

Witness how the heat of the kundalini breaks through the blockage at muladhara, the root chakra and opens the knot of Brahma.

70

Continue breathing and pay attention as the energy starts to ascend in 3½ cycles up the shushmana, the central channel, and creates brilliance inside the sushmana channel. It looks like a brilliant silver cord from the muladhara chakra to the throat chakra.

Relax the breath.

Softly chant the mantra: 'Wahe Guru' and continue to chant as you vibrate the mantra in the sushmana channel, continue to chant and see the sushmana channel as a silver cord from the root chakra to the throat chakra.

> *Wahe Guru, Wahe Guru Wahe Guru, Wahe Guru,*
> *Wahe Guru, Wahe Guru, Wahe Guru, Wahe Guru*

Once the silver cord is awakened relax into long deep breathing again.

On the exhalation, apply uddhiyana bandh, diaphragm lock and notice how this moves the kundalini through the fourth chakra, opening the knot of Vishnu. Continue to apply this bandha on the exhalation until you sit with a heart as wide as the world.

Relax for a few breaths.

On the exhalation apply Jalandhar bandh, neck lock, recognize how this bandha guides the kundalini through its final blockage at the throat chakra.

Continue to only breathe long and deep, and pay attention as the heat from the kundalini causes the pineal to transmit a beam of radiation and projects it to the pituitary. Now the pituitary projects impulses, creating visions of color at the third eye increasing the potential to be more intuitive.

Breathe.

This activation of the pineal and pituitary causes their union at the third eye. Observe the golden cord — the gate that links the pineal and pituitary glands to the crown chakra— awaken.

The kundalini now rises to the pineal gland, the tenth gate—the seat of the soul—permeating the cells of the brain and the chakra centers in the brain.

As the knot of Shiva opens, witness how the thousand-petaled lotus, the crown chakra filled with kundalini energy turns and the kundalini pours from the crown chakra back down to the root chakra. Observe how each of the chakras turns up to receive the kundalini and each chakra opens fully as the kundalini descends.

Breathe into your brilliance.

Inhale deeply and hold the breath, do these 3 times and then relax.

Sat Nam!

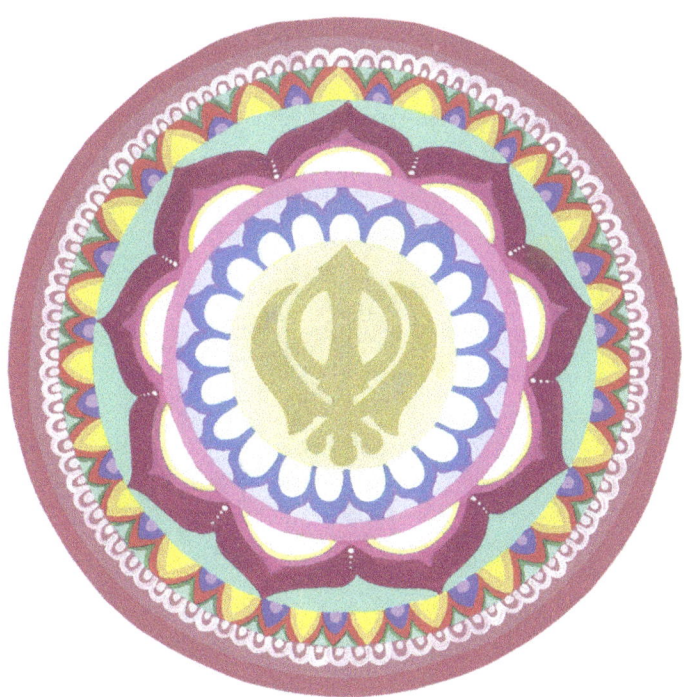

CHAPTER 5
THE GUIDE – INTRODUCTION

There is One. Central Biorhythm from which all of creation,
Prakirti, manifests.
Prakirti is highly organized and predictable according to Universal
laws.
These laws are observable within and without.
Life requires voltae, prana, and a magnetic field
– an aura to live and Thrive.

REVIEW

Life creates a magnetic field, and when the energy is contained it attracts to itself. Self-containment happens when the yogi consciously harmonizes the energy flow through the electrical system of the first 6 Chakras. The 7th body can then create a contained magnetic field, which in turn amplifies the brilliance of the subtle bodies. The magnetic field maintains the homeostasis of the electrical system, and protects the identity by containing the five tattvas.

This model, of an environment with a person at its center enclosed by various light sources, is actually a pretty good, however poetic description of a psyche. This sense of a being at the center of an illuminated field is at the core of the classical yogic view. The aim then, is to recognize the self at the center and to understand and identify with this light-pattern. Again, that a pattern exists is a fact, and the rest—that is, the process of identifying with that pattern—is a matter of interpretation.

We identify the self- sensory human being as someone attuned to the light patterns, the brilliance of the soul's expression by means of the 10 aspects of the psyche. As a self-sensory being, you practice to be more aware to ease or dis-ease, and gradually your ability to observe where you are out of balance will become more acute. Once in yoga class we spoke to how yoga and meditation make you more sensitive and a student asked: "Why would I want to become more sensitive?" The question made a lot of sense seeing how many people work very hard to desensitize, to go "numb". Yet, it is a well-known fact that in order to feel the bliss and joy, you have to also feel the pain and the sorrow. It is all the expression of life, two sides of the same coin, and you can't have one without the other. You will learn to read your feelings, your sensations, and use them as your guidance system. Those feelings that cause you pain are only your indicators as to where you can deepen and open up more to Universal energy. Being sensitive will allow you to be more aware of the world you are creating. You create by giving your attention, just like watering your garden. It's not only the flowers which start to grow, it's also the weeds. Knowing that water makes everything in your garden grow makes you pay more attention as to what you are watering. Your feelings attune you to what you are focusing your prana on, so you can start to water and grow only those thoughts and projections, which you intend to.

The guide can give direction and clarity in this observation process and later on in this chapter, there are further descriptions for each aspect listed in the guide. Chapter 6 outlines intentional actions, which you can do to bring greater harmony to the expression of that aspect. Yogic practices and foods will be sprinkled in other parts of the book as they have such a significant impact on the vibratory patterning of the body.

BALANCE

As with the chakras and Ten Bodies, the idea is that balance, shunia, has its own reward. An energy produced in the state of ease is qualitatively different than the kind produced in a state of dis-ease. The premise is that when we use the guide and identify with a pattern of imbalance, where ease is not the pervading frequency, that the environment for dis-ease is present. Energy is never stagnant, it is always creating ease or dis-ease, expansion or contraction. Our purpose in sharing this information is to give you the understanding of how to keep your energy flowing in patterns, which create health (ease).

In old China it was understood that health was our most natural and balanced expression. Doctors would get paid as long as the patient was healthy, and as soon as the patient got ill, payment would be withheld because the doctor was not doing their job. Imagine how our society would change if we paid for the state of health instead of the state of disease!

THE GUIDE

This is how the guide works: on the left side are the observations of possible imbalances. On the right side of the chart, there are correspondent healthy intentional actions that can be adopted in order to support health (ease). Each line therefore is it's whole own story. It contains the questions, the pain points and the answers, the intentional actions.

General application of the guide
- Identify an imbalance.
- Observe if it appears in more then one place on that line.
- Identify intentional actions.
- Apply them to your life.

The information in the observation columns are from various healing modalities, which identify the balance or imbalance of the energy. Descriptions for each of the observations are provided to give you more information.

The Intentional Action part of the chart consists of actions you can do to regain a sense of ease, and to experience deeper harmony in your life. At the top of the chart it also indicates where the information in the column comes from: Western tradition, Chinese or Yoga. These systems are circular and sometimes overlap and also can at times feel different from what perhaps one discipline has taught.

The chart is a guide and only that. It is not the be all and end all of healing by any means. Our own method is to look at an issue from a western anatomical and a physiological perspective first. Then, we use this guide to see if the issue can be approached at a causal level prior to medication or surgical intervention. We have found in most cases that this is a more effective and less costly approach, yet there are instances in which the western way is the only option.

The chart as a guide can be used for the purposes of awareness. From it, the casual reader will gain some understanding and a doctor will see that the energetic patterns of the body are steady and predictable. A seeker however, will put the data into practice. A committed spiritual discipline will provoke various signals, such as thoughts, emotions or bodily sensations. Using the chart as a roadmap, it is possible for the yogi to observe and understand the channels through which these signals are conveyed, and with deep observation, the content of what is being conveyed.

DR. GURUCHANDER

Taking a look at my approach as a physician, there is one outcome that I always seek in treating my patients and when teaching yoga students: to make them calmer, to move their energy from dis-ease to ease. This can be especially challenging when assessing health issues. Just as the seeker, in learning and adopting new perspectives, can sometimes be overwhelmed with information, the peaceful feeling I aim to instill is tenuous. A patient can sometimes be discouraged just because they have an issue. And a yogi can become frustrated because it is impossible to always see the path ahead. Even when consistently engaged in their spiritual practice, the lack of knowing what is next can undermine the passion to continue with a practice. However, just as the patient speaks to the doctor, the yogi develops a discourse between body, mind, and soul. In the course of these processes, both the patient and the yogi learn trust, and that trust builds the ability to recognize and dwell in that serenity.

This kind of serenity, the kind that can be practiced, pervades even in the face of that which is unexpected. The possibility of a supreme ease exists. It is actual and embodied in the life of a yogi.

As a physician, I look at my patients, who are by definition without ease, and therefore in "dis-ease." This word is used in Western medical circles in a very specific way, but here it means any lack of harmony within one or more of the systems presented. These are the imbalances the guide will indicate.

CHANGE

Transformation means positive change and change, as President Kennedy said, is the only constant. A spiritual seeker accepts continuous transformation as the truth and commits to significant and ongoing change. This process means going through various stages of being as something-other-than-enlightened first, which isn't always comfortable. In philosophy, these are what are known as "differences of degree." In order to live as a truly and absolutely free being, there must be a "difference in kind." To put it simply, a person with one specific quality of being must become another kind of person with a totally different set of qualities attendant to the new state of being.

This means a whole new set of habits, the most important of which are yoga and meditation. These provide the moments for self-reflection to observe the relative serenity in every aspect of life. With brilliance as the standard, the process of self-examination will ultimately lead to ease.

The process of change, which the guide calls for, appears to be both passive in the observations and active in the application of the intentional actions. Observation can be most clear when in a state of Shunia. The stillness provides a higher vantage point from which to observe patterns of imbalance and opportunities for healing.

We see our experience on this planet as an opportunity to take opposites and create something entirely new, from the amalgamation of the polarities into a new harmonic balance.

The guide offers more light on the journey, more awareness of how to deepen into a state of shunia. The word on the "spiritual street" is that our natural state is one of ease and bliss, that happiness is actually our birthright, and that we work really hard to dis-allow this. We say it's time to claim our joy!

HABITS

While the guide will help to make the signals more readily interpretable, with genuine commitment, there may be challenges that will humble the student. This is easily understood as we move from self-sabotaging and destructive habits to new, calm inducing ones. After all, if the intention is to change, there will certainly be instances where old habits are repeated. Just like walking on a beach with each step forward, you also slide back in the sand just a bit. Even changing something simple will sometimes provoke a serious mental reaction. Don't worry when this happens. Just learn from it. The guide assists in this learning process. By understanding which signals come from where, these tough moments can become deeply healing and opportunities for sincere self-assessment.

The most important habit is a mental one. Hold the intention and commit all your energy to that intention. What does brilliance or enlightenment mean to you? What will it look like once you're there? Take the time, right now, to be clear about these particulars. Ask yourself, "What is the depth of my commitment?" If you can honestly declare that enlightenment is attainable, the waves of distraction will be less intense. You can see it as already done and therefore practice it with ease. The attitude of the yogi is to rise above the drama in every situation of life. That stated conviction would engender the attitude to facilitate and initiate the new habits to support all the bodies' systems, keeping the body and mind directed toward Purest Potential with joy and ease.

Every disciplined practice to elevate the 10 bodies changes the effectiveness of all things forever, because everything corresponds to the polarity of the magnetic field of an ever-

78

expanding universe. The energetic patterns of our habits can't be changed by emotions or sentiments, but only when the actual force of the magnetic field around them supports the different voltage of a higher intention. Life is an interrelated, interconnected magnetic field.

Enjoy your exploration of the guide as it provides a way to observe your relationship to this interrelated, interconnected magnetic field and all which that implies...

The following chart is available for download on the Purest Potential Website: www.purestpotential.com/thank-you-book

Observation Part 1

Yoga	Astrology	Chinese	Yoga	Yoga	Chinese
Bodies & Chakras	Sign	Meridian	Tattva	Tattva Projection	Tissue
1	Gemini	Stomach	Earth	Greed	Muscles
1	Cancer	Spleen & Pancreas	Earth	Greed	Muscles
2	Libra	Bladder	Water	Lust	Bones, Head Hair
2	Scorpio	Kidneys	Water	Lust	Bones, Head Hair
3	Aquarius	Gallbladder	Fire	Anger	Tendons
3	Pisces	Liver	Fire	Anger	Tendons
4	Aries	Lungs	Air	Attachment	Skin, Body Hair
4	Taurus	Large Intestine	Air	Attachment	Skin, Body Hair
5	Leo	Heart	Ether	Pride	Vessels
5	Virgo	Small Intestine	Ether	Pride	Vessels
6	Sagittarius	Nervous System			Nerve Tissue
6	Capricorn	Glandular System			Glandular Tissue
7					
8					
9					
10					
11					

Observation Part 2

Yoga	Chinese	Chinese	Yoga	Yoga	Chinese
	Body Part	Location	Sense	Organ	Negative
1	Arms / Shoulders	Outside Leg	Smell	Nose	Exclusive
1	Breasts	Inside Leg	Smell	Nose	Inflexible
2	Lower Back	Outside Leg	Taste	Tongue	Pessimistic
2	Reproductive Organs	Inside Leg	Taste	Tongue	Fearful / Worried
3	Ankles	Outside Leg	Sight	Eyes	Intolerance
3	Feet	Inside Leg	Sight	Eyes	Anger
4	Head	Outside Arm	Touch	Skin	No Understanding
4	Neck	Inside Arm	Touch	Skin	Unsteady
5	Spine	Inside Arm	Speech	Ears	Coward
5	Abdomen	Outside Arm	Speech	Ears	Critical
6	Hips	Inside Arm	ESP	Nerves	Nervous
6	Knees	Outside Arm	ESP	Glands	Commotional
7					
8					
9					
10					
11					

Intentional Action Part 1

Yoga	Chinese	Yoga	Western	Chinese	Chinese	Yoga
	Time of Aggravation & Action	Mudra	Cell Salt	Taste	Food Color	Affirmation
1	7am – 9am	Buddhi Mudra	Kali Mur	Sweet	Yellow	I Create
1	9am – 11am	Buddhi Mudra	Calc Fluor	Sweet	Yellow	I Create
2	3pm – 5pm	Venus Lock	Nat Phos	Salty	Black	I Connect
2	5pm – 7pm	Venus Lock	Calc Sulph	Salty	Black	I Connect
3	11pm – 1am	Chander Mudra	Nat Mur	Sour	Green	I Give Hope
3	1am – 3am	Chander Mudra	Ferr Phos	Sour	Green	I Give Hope
4	3am – 5am	Prayer Pose at Heart	Kali Phos	Pungent	White	I Serve
4	5am – 7am	Prayer Pose at Heart	Nat Sulph	Pungent	White	I Serve
5	11am – 1pm	Buddhi Mudra	Mag Phos	Bitter	Red	I Teach
5	1pm – 3pm	Buddhi Mudra	Kali Sulph	Bitter	Red	I Teach
6	7pm – 9pm	Ganesh Mudra	Silica	Astringent	Clear	I Focus
6	9pm – 11pm	Ganesh Mudra	Calc Phos	Astringent	Clear	I Focus
7		Arms 60 Degrees			Violet	I Contain
8		Gian Mudra			White	I Am Courageous
9		Shuni Mudra			Silver	I Am a Master
10		Surya Mudra			Gold	I Am Radiant
11		Yogi Mudra				Unto Infinity

Intentional Action Part 2

Yoga	Yoga	Yoga	Yoga	Chinese
	Naad Yoga	Tattva Balancing	Action	Positive Emotion
1	Mul Mantra	Heart Over Head	Be Creative	All Embracing
1	Mul Mantra	Heart Over Head	Be Creative	Flexible
2	Adi Shakti	Long to Belong	Connect with Self	Optimistic
2	Adi Shakti	Long to Belong	Connect with Self	Fearless
3	Hari Har	Devil or Divine	Be Positive	Tolerance
3	Hari Har	Devil or Divine	Be Positive	Friendly
4	RaMaDaSa	Cup of Prayer	Be Compassionate	Understanding
4	RaMaDaSa	Cup of Prayer	Be Compassionate	Steady
5	I am, I am	Teacher, Balance	Chant	Brave
5	I am, I am	Teacher, Balance	Chant	Uplifting
6	Ong		Meditate	Calm
6	Ong		Meditate	Devotional
7	Ma			Contain
8	Wahe Guru		Pranayam	Courage
9	Sat Nam			Mastery
10	Gobinda			Radiant
11	Fateh			Unto Infinity

CHAPTER 6
OBSERVATIONS AND INTENTIONAL ACTIONS

We do it through meditation. Your constitution consists of five tattvas, seven chakras, and 10 bodies. Life is best lived when these are all balanced as they are all interested. We create balance through yoga, meditation, conscious lifestyle choices and chanting.

We will follow the lay out of the guide moving from left to right, from observations to intentional actions.

BODIES & CHAKRAS
According to Kundalini Yoga

As energetic entities, each chakra and each of the Ten Bodies is the energetic container for samskaras and karmic patterns specific to that location. What follows is an outline of these patterns as imbalances that can be observed as well as, corrected by practicing the specific yoga kriya for the body in question (see kriyas at the end of the book).

1st Chakra & Soul Body

If 1st Chakra is imbalanced you might notice: hemorrhoids, constipation, sciatica, low back pain, stomach, spleen, and/or pancreas problems.

If 1st Body is imbalanced you might notice: you come from your head instead of your heart, feel stuck, constipated in life, unable to act, can't get grounded on earth, people call you spaced out, insecure, feel unsafe, too dependent on others, lack of creativity.

When it is balanced you might notice: That you feel you have a strong foundation, grounded to earth, you feel safe and secure, you can trust in yourself easily, you have the ability to stand alone, to provide for yourself, you have a good balance between dependence and independence, you are creative.

Intentional Action: go on silence, stop thinking and do something creative instead, hand flashes to stimulate creative flow. This is how to do hand flashes: hands in fists, open and close fists and alternate thumb in and out as you open and close fists. Take an art course, color mandalas, write your epitaph, eat no more than 2 cups of food per meal, eat less sweets, inhale and exhale three times and then put hands under left rib and pull stomach down towards the navel.

Yoga: crow pose, chair pose, body drops, frog pose, double leg front stretch, lie on stomach kick buttocks with feet, all 1st body yoga kriyas and meditations from our books.

Food: Take chlorophyll and some form of pro-biotics to keep elimination regular, triphala, yellow squash, corn, ripe banana, papaya, aloe vera, drink warm water.

2nd Chakra & Negative Mind Body

If 2nd Chakra is imbalanced you might notice: uterine and ovarian problems, sexual dysfunction, vaginal problems, pelvic pain, prostate problems, kidney and/or bladder problems.

If 2nd Body is imbalanced you might notice: You avoid relationships, feel sexually repressed, vacillate between feeling connected and disconnected, feel unable to have successful interactions with others, deny yourself pleasure, excess sexual fantasies, fear of abandonment, experience emotion becoming commotion in many areas of life, dis-obey your inner guidance and create more polarization/Karma.

When balanced you might notice: an emotional life where you can express your opinions, balanced feelings, connectedness to Self, healthy sensuality and sexuality, ability to experience pleasure, feel very contained in your actions and with your decisions in life, easily discourse and obey your inner voice the light of your soul, you live your Dharma.

Intentional Action: chant mantra: 'I AM, I AM'; go for a run; mind follows the breath so do any pranayama especially 2 part breath, take action vs. worry, be in water, compose your absolute "No" list. Your list of your deal breakers for every area of life. For example: I will not be with someone who lies to me.

Yoga: Frog pose, cobra, cat-cow, pelvic lifts, spinal rock with knees apart, butterfly, all 2nd body yoga kriyas and meditations from our books, all Venus kriyas.

Food: Drink cucumber juice, black chickpea/garbanzo beans, black beans, drink 12 oz. cucumber juice for 40 days with good food, drink corn silk tea.

3rd Chakra & Positive Mind Body

When 3rd Chakra is imbalanced you might notice: difficulty with digestion and absorption, liver problems, headaches, feet pain, eye dysfunction and deterioration of vision, all pain symptoms, gallbladder problems.

If the 3rd Body is imbalanced you might notice: outbursts of anger, intolerance, issues with power and authority, fear of success, depression, unable to see hope or give yourself hope, can't foresee the positive outcomes from your own actions in calculating the future, judgmental of others.

Balanced you might notice: healthy assertiveness, confidence, can digest the events of life in a positive light, healthy physical digestion, strong will power, enjoy being the power, to be an expansive light, easy to be the authority in groups, manifest successful life patterns, hope giver, bliss seeking and realizing, see all others as equals, apply your will to manifest own future and help others to do the same, express frustration with calm.

Intentional Action: exercise more, create balance between work and play, record yourself reading positive affirmations and listen to them when you sleep, take a martial arts class, set goals and achieve them.

Yoga: stretch pose, bow pose, double leg lifts, breath of fire, locust pose, sat kriya, all 3rd body yoga kriyas and meditations from our books, exercise more, walk 3 miles daily and swing your arms.

Food: grapefruit, greens, lemons, yogurt, chlorophyll, raw turmeric with yogurt, apple cider vinegar to maintain your metabolism, follow this Ayurvedic advice for proper metabolism: divide your stomach into four parts, 1/4 for air, 1/4 for water, 1/4 for food, and 1/4 for appetizer (salad or green vegetable), eat white daikon radish.

4th Chakra & Neutral Mind Body

When 4rd Chakra is imbalanced you might notice: breast, chest, heart, lung and large intestine problems, breathing difficulties.

When the 4th Body is imbalanced you might notice: Inability to be neutral, always have an opinion about everything, unable to live unless in polarity, overly attached to almost everything, sadness, poor listening skills.

When balanced: joy, easy to give and receive, compassion, empathy, forgiveness, love, devotion, kindness, consideration, healing, a yogi, great deep listener, compassionate, deep breather, get second wind easily in physical activities.

Intentional action: Communicate what is 'right' not what you want, bhakti yoga, wear white clothes, Puja/worship to the Guru; the source which guides you to your own light; not as a person but as a representation of your own neutral mind as a consciousness, devotional dance, get trained to become a mediator or negotiator, devotional chanting.

Yoga: side twists, spine flex, ego eradicator, all arm exercises, cobra, bow pose, bridge pose, yoga mudra, pranayam, kirtan kriya, cross crawl exercises, all 4th body yoga kriyas and meditations from our books.

Food: eat white foods, onions, cauliflower, garlic, ginger, rice etc.

5th Chakra & "Physical" Body

When the 5th Chakra is imbalanced you might notice: throat, speech, ear, heart, small intestine and neck problems.

When the 5th Body is imbalanced you might notice: inability to voice your feelings, poor communication skills, unable to sacrifice your time for others, fear of teaching and of being in front of others and giving instruction, poor physical health, workaholic, lazy, cant express what your destiny/intention is.

Balanced: express your destiny, easy to speak your truth, easy to communicate, great listener, teacher, ability to command through speech, speak things into being, ability to respond with balance, balanced life i.e. sacrifices for others and balances with needs for own well being.

Intentional Actions: chant, mantra yoga, aerobic exercise for at least 30 minutes daily, gentle intestinal cleansing, use Purest Potential neck block, speak at public speaking events, set up daily habits to maintain a balance between work and play, practice kaurie kriya.

Yoga: shoulder stand, plow pose, cobra, neck rolls, nose to knees while on back, cat cow, buddhi mudra: with each hand hold tips of pinky and thumb together and chant: 'RA RA RA RA, MA MA MA MA, RAMA RAMA RAMA RAMA, SATANAMA', Breath of Fire, all 5th body yoga kriyas and meditations from our books.

Food: Chilies, lecithin.

6th Chakra & The Arc Line Body

The 6th Body is about projection/expansion and protection.

This expansion manifests in:
*The 7th Body as the aura.
*The 8th Body as the Magnetic Field.
*The 9th Body as the Etheric Body.
*The 10th Body as the Circumvent Force.

Imbalances in the 6th Chakra might show up as: glandular imbalances, vision problems, learning disabilities, and problems with nervous and glandular system, weak immune system.

Imbalances in the 6th Body might show up as: confusion, inability to focus, over-intellectualizing, inconsistency in mood and behavior, unable to manifest your projects, cannot access intuitive guidance in life.

Balanced: intuition, clairvoyance, ability to visualize, wisdom, insight, concentration, ability to focus, understanding your life purpose, see beyond duality, integration, able to hold a mental projection, maintain goals, care and support for all life, prayerful projection, clear sense of justice, natural meditator, protection of self and others.

Intentional Actions: create a vision board, see what needs to be seen vs. what is, hear Truth with third eye and never forget it, intentional prayer which creates a vibratory effect which goes into the Infinite creative psyche, express I am I am, let the hair under your arms grow because according to Ayurveda the armpits are the balance point between the sympathetic and parasympathetic nervous systems, and your eyebrows and eyelashes are the 'messengers' to the nervous system, do intestinal cleansing, clear your space with Palo Santo or sage, set up an altar and bow before it every morning.

Yoga: focus at 3rd eye point, archer pose, baby pose, sit on heels inhale and exhale bow down to floor, yoga mudra, all 6th body yoga kriyas and meditations from our books, Breath of Fire, alternate nostril breathing blends the prana and apana and gives control at the 6th chakra, Sat Kriya, shoulder stand 11 min daily, Tratakam meditation, chant Wahe Guru.

Food: celery, bananas, cucumber, yogi tea, onion, garlic, ginger, 16 oz. of celery juice, oatmeal water: soak 1/4 cup of oats in 4 cups of water for 20 min and then drink, yogi tea with ginger, vitamin B complex, sesame seeds, eat fruits that begin with a p, pears, papayas etc.

7th Chakra & Aura Body

Imbalances in the 7th Chakra might show up as: sleep problems, susceptibility to the flu and colds.

Imbalances in the 7th Body might show up as: can't screen out negative events or thoughts after talking to those you care about, feel it's your destiny to fix other people's problems, lay awake at night ruminating about the cure for other people's problems, vulnerable in crowd's and hard to stay true to oneself, no boundaries or sense of being self-contained, no boundaries from physical invasion and protection, insecure and feel unsafe.

Balanced: Secure as Self so that you feel sovereign, safe in identity as a light of the soul, very contained person, show mercy to all life, love Self, doesn't feel responsible to heal others and teach others how to heal themselves.

Intentional Action: increase the ways in which you nurture yourself, meditation on crown of the head, chanting/singing, journal observations of how the aura reflects your mental habits, visualize a 9 foot aura extending out in all directions from your body like an envelope around you then chant 'AD GURAY NAMEH' and visualize the first quarter of this envelope radiant, then chant 'JUGAD GURAY NAMEH' and visualize the second quarter radiant, chant 'SAT GURAY NAMEH' visualize the 3rd quarter radiant, then chant 'SIRI GURU DAVAY NAMEH' and visualize the 4th quarter radiant.

Yoga: ego eradicator, focus on tip of nose, all 7th body yoga kriyas and meditations from our books, chant 'MA' mantra.

Food: balanced organic foods.

8th Pranic Body

An imbalanced 8th Body might show up as: constricted diaphragm resulting in shallow rapid breathing, fear patterns, always tired, unable to start and or finish projects, tendency towards self-destruction, a dare devil.

Balanced: energy, fearlessness, self-initiates: i.e. generate, organize, and deliver projects.

Intentional Action: celestial communication, asanas to balance the pelvic bone which then can encourage the breathing power of the pranic body, long deep breathing from navel, pranayam to look more brilliant and "shinier", don't use make up, all aerobic exercises, sing, Gutka paintra* 11 min daily, blow up a balloon 10x daily, learn a form of energy healing ex. Sat Nam Rasayan.

Yoga: triangle pose, archer pose, arm exercises, horse stance with Breath of Fire, windmills, any meditation with an intention for healing, Breath of Fire, any pranayam, move from camel pose to baby pose, all 8th body yoga kriyas and meditations from our books, 1 minute breath meditation.

9th Subtle Body

An imbalanced 9th Body might show up as: naïve and easily fooled, unintentionally crude or rough in speech or behavior, experience restlessness.

A balanced 9th Body might show up as: powerful calmness, great finesse, see beyond the obvious, learn and master situations easily, subtlety, mastery.

Intentional action: wear nice clothes and jewelry, Japanese tea ceremony, Tai Chi, shavasana during the day, practice walking meditations.

Yoga Asanas: Any meditation or yoga set done for 1000 days, all 9th body yoga kriyas and meditations from our books.

Food: Practice Bhoj Kriya, bless food before eating.

10th Radiant Body

An imbalanced 10th Body might show up as: No sophistication in actions, afraid to take leadership roles, doesn't like to stand out ever, dresses down.

A balanced 10th Body might show up as: exert a magnetic presence and command vs. demand respect, have great strength, determination and stamina, give 110%, radiance, nobility, royal courage, can neutralize own negativity.

Intentional Action: Archer pose 11 minutes each side, grow all your hair, assess your possessions and only keep those you really love, dress up like royalty.

Yoga: all 10th body yoga kriyas and meditations from our books.

Food: cucumber juice, corn silk tea, silica from foods.

11th Body

An Imbalanced 11th Body might show up as: narrow mindedness, small thinking, and lack of future vision, dumbing down.

A balanced 11th Body might show up as: futuristic thinking with big vision, help all to grow and become vast.

Intentional Action: go through a process to declare your past complete, acupuncture, healing sound gong immersions, early morning yoga practice, DON'T dumb down, practice patience, get more flexible, create a 10 body check in list and review daily.

Yoga: all kriyas for the 11th Body from our books.

Food: kitcheree, and foods that contain all 6 tastes in balance.

ASTROLOGICAL SIGN

For the purposes of Purest Potential, it is important to recognize that the various forms of astrology Chinese, Vedic and Western; not only share their foundations and general outlook, but also link directly into the bodily systems explored in this book. Specifically, Western astrology and Chinese medicine link the Sun Sign directly to the meridians and thus to the chakras. Further, the Chinese system identifies these patterns of light as they occur during the course of the day. You will find this represented in the 'times' column in the chart.

Yogis believe that we choose our time of birth consciously in order to assist us in learning and elevating our life lessons. Each sign has some tendency that can be exaggerated, the focus here is to create awareness so that you can transform and elevate your imbalanced tendencies into strengths. When someone is born under the aspect of these magnetic field energies, created from the constellation of the stars, it affects the water, which forms 70% of the body. The information in the guide can help you identify the negative tendencies and give solutions for reversing the patterns. Your opportunity is to overcome the tendencies.

There are definitely lessons to be learned in exploring these tendencies. Self-examination is, after all, absolutely part of self-development and transformation. Knowing astrology is not necessary, but if there is an interest in exploring this field, especially given the nature of application to healing offered, then there is one thing that must be kept in mind: recognize that the pattern of the stars at the time of birth is in the past. The circumstances of this life differ from those before birth. This observation offers everyone the opportunity to transcend the pattern in a given astrological reading and to rewrite destiny. Looking at it clearly, astrology then only speaks to the lessons the soul came to learn this lifetime.

What we need to be aware of in regards to each of the astrological signs is the predominant energy circuits that may create dis-ease for you. The astrological signs are actually the same as the main 12 meridians. These meridians come in pairs that balance each other along the spine at energy vortexes, the chakras. In each pair one meridian spins clockwise and one counter clockwise. The yogi consciously chooses a lifestyle that will assure a delicate energetic balance between the two meridians, or nadis, at the chakra point, plus strengthen the magnetic field to hold this balance during a full day of input from our senses.

How the Planets Relate to the 10 Bodies

BODIES	PLANET	YOGIC EXPRESSION
1st	MERCURY	HEART OVER HEAD
2nd	VENUS	LONGING TO BELONG
3rd	MOON	DEVIL OR DIVINE
4th	MARS	CUP OF PRAYER
5th	JUPITER	HALF BALANCE
6th	SATURN	PERSON AT PRAYER
7th	URANUS	PLATFORM OF ELEVATION
8th	NEPTUNE	FINITE TO INFINITE
9th	PLUTO	GOD AND BLESSINGS
10th	SUN	REACH FOR INFINITY
11TH EMBODIMENT	UNTO INFINITY	UNTO INFINITY

MERIDIANS

The flow of prana through the meridians provides an observable pattern, which tells us if there is harmony or dis-harmony in those energy channels.

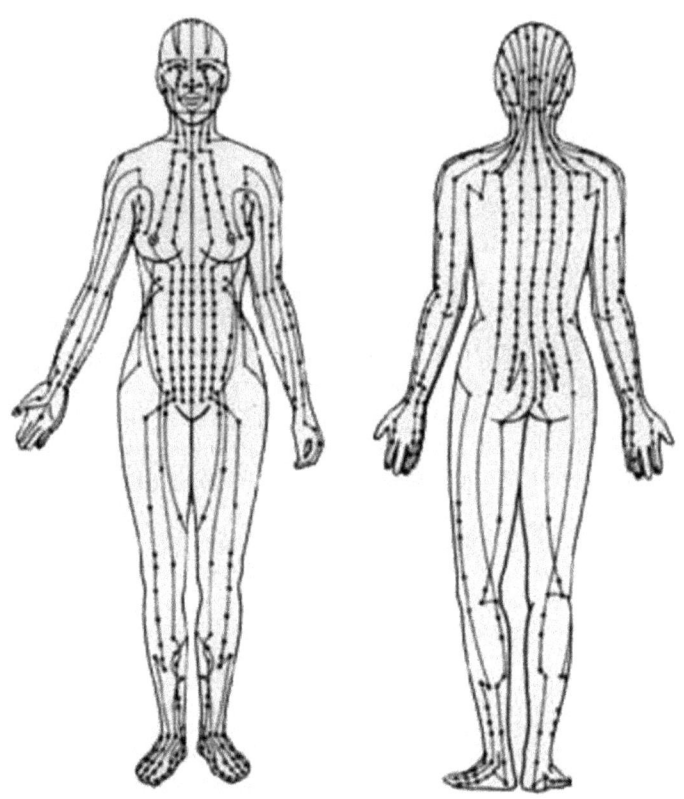

TATTVA

The magnetic structure of life is created from the combinations of the five tattvas, or elements: earth, water, fire, air and ether. Each tattva has a positive and a negative projection, which is discussed under the Tattva Projection column.

In all ancient philosophy, including both Eastern and pre-Socratic Western philosophy, the five elements were the primary way in which the unity of all manifestation was understood. Since everything within human experience is made up of the same stuff, there has always been a natural affinity between people and nature, the heavens and the earth. In time, the Western tradition dropped this way of thinking. However Chinese medicine and Ayurveda, the Indian science of life, maintain these traditional views in their core principles and practices.

The basic approach of the ancients was intuitive. For example: that which consists mostly of earth tends to naturally fall toward the earth. Similarly, fire which rises naturally was said to reside in the heavens, its home in the stars. Different schools of thought on these matters arranged the elements in differing orders, but the principle of their organization was always the same, from the least subtle to the most: earth, water, fire, air and ether.

Humans were of particular interest to these ancients, since they recognized that they were alone in observing these subtleties. So they assigned the elements various places to reside within the human body as you can see in the guide. These are the chakras and their arrangement in elemental order ascending subtlety. First Chakra: earth. Second Chakra: water, Third Chakra: fire. Fourth Chakra: air. Fifth Chakra: ether. It was thought to be a microcosm for the macrocosm, our whole universe.

These elements can be adjusted when imbalances occur:

- To balance the earth element, which represents solidity, your karma and ego, make sure your elimination is effective.
- To balance the water element and invoke the quality to flow through anything, in meditation apply the mudra: Venus lock.
- To balance the fire element practice stretch pose.
- To balance the air element, which has the quality to reflect a temperature of either hot or cold and not become it, use alternate nostril breathing.
- To balance the ether element, which has the quality to be like the sky, unchanging and the same for everyone, inhale through the curled tongue and exhale through the nose.

Keeping all the elements in balance is a powerful tool to maintain a state of health.

TATTVA PROJECTION

TATTVA	NEGATIVE TATTVA PROJECTION ~Finite self~	POSITIVE TATTVA PROJECTION ~Infinite Self~
Earth	Greed for self	Greed for Self
Water	Lust for self	Lust for Self
Fire	Anger from self	Anger when not with Self
Air	Attachment to self	Attachment to Self
Ether	Pride in Self	Pride in the Oneness with Self

The negative expressions of the Tattvas can be observed as destructive patterns of behavior and can be changed into the positive expression of that Tattva.

- The negative projections of the Tattvas are the Bhavs.
- The positive projections are the Prabhu- Bhavs.

Behavior of the Tattvas

Destructive patterns of behavior are related to negative expression of the five tattvas: ether, air, water, fire and earth.

Earth (lobh) pertains to greed and desires for recognition and territory: **Fire** (krodh) to anger, rough language and neurotic behavior: **Water** (kam) to sensuality and lust; and **Air** (Moh) to my-ness, identity and power.

The latter is because air contains life-giving energy (prana), and it therefore gives you your identity. There are two aspects of identity in life, I-ness and my-ness.

Lastly, the tattva of ether (ahangkar) pertains to we (hum) – pride, false ego, negative id, boasting and lack of humility.

The above behaviors reflect the bhavs or negative side of the tattvas. The tattva bhavs must be channeled to positive expression, prabhu bhavs. If you have pride, be proud to be holy, righteous, graceful and conscious. If you have attachment and identity, identify yourself with goodness, grace, sweetness and sacrifice. If you have anger, be angry at your neuroses, consume your negativities, falsehood and lower nature.

Use your power to be serviceful, graceful and kind against adverse and ungraceful environments. If you want to create a relationship, create it with your higher consciousness and divinity. If you are in your negative id or ego, remember that you are a creature who belongs to the Creator. A negative ego is the biggest disease, but it holds its own solutions. If you transfer the ego from passion to compassion, you will become divine.

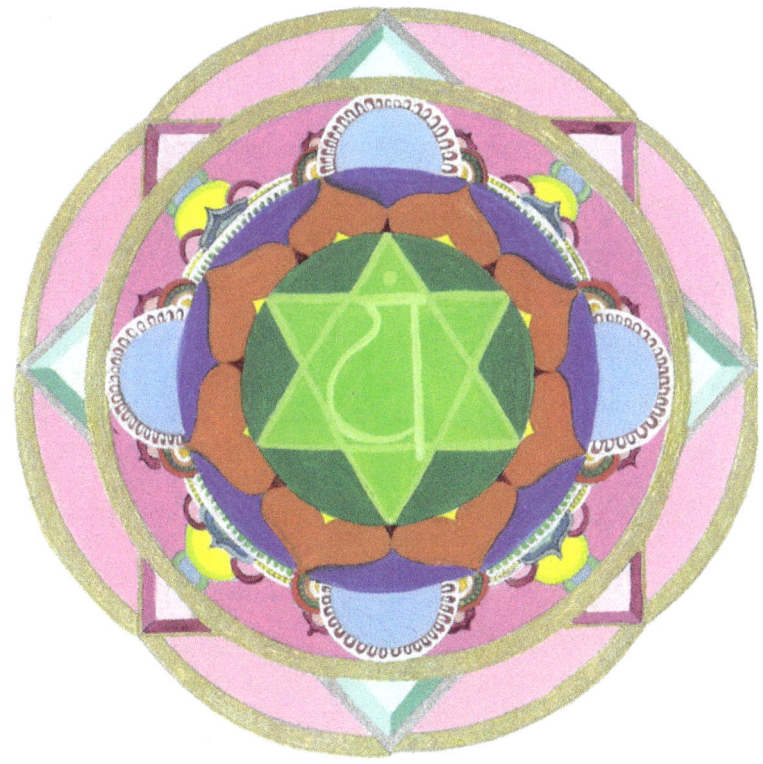

Practice to channel the Bhavs into Prabhu Bhavs.

They each hold their own solution!

TATTVA	BHAV	PRABHU BHAV
EARTH	Greed, desire for recognition, desire for territory	Be greedy to identify with goodness, grace, sweetness, creativity and sacrifice
WATER	Sensuality, lust	Lust for connectedness with your higher consciousness and divinity
FIRE	Anger, rough language, neurotic behavior	Be angry at your neurosis, consume your negativities, falsehood and lower nature, achieve bliss with Self
AIR	My-ness, identity, power, attachment	Be attached to use your power to do seva, use power to be kind in adverse environments, be attached to Self
ETHER	Pride, false ego, boasting and lack of humility	Be proud to be sacred, righteous, graceful, conscious

TISSUES- the connective structural element of the body
- Muscles
- Vessels
- Bones
- Nerves
- Glandular Tissue

The first indicator of energetic imbalance is often an irritation or inflammation of the different kinds of tissues in the body. From the yogic perspective all disease is a manifestation of anger, which causes a reduction of the flow of prana. The tissues have various but specific roles to play in the body's basic function. In their operation, we observe disease, which comes from samskaras and karmas. For healing to take place, there must be a reduction of anger/ inflammation, which then increases the flow of prana to all the tissues listed above. Our lifestyle choices develop the habits, which provide the psyche the means to balance itself. Physical or mental discomfort can become a clue. The experience of inflammation in the tissues guides us to determine which of the 10 Bodies is out of balance.

Each Tissue Represents a Tattva

Earth	Muscles
Water	Bones
Fire	Blood vessels
Air	Nerves
Ether	Glands

BODY PART

Body Part provides clues to patterns. For example, if there is pain in the head it is a clue that there could be an issue with the internal representation of the lung. Any of the Body Parts experiencing pain or inflammation could possibly be a clue to a meridian dysfunction. When we reduce anger then we create ease and decrease inflammation.

By observing the body parts you can know which of the 10 Bodies is out of balance.

1st	Triceps, Latissmus dorsi, earth
2nd	Psoas, water
3rd	Abdominal muscles, wood
4th	Diaphragm, metal
5th	Neck and shoulder muscles, fire
6th	Gluteus Maximus
7th	Weak spleen meridian, triceps
8th	Diaphragm weakness
9th	Lack of muscular grace
10th	Overall coordination and synchronization
11th	Mastery of the entire physical realm

When we find spasm in the muscle, according to Dr. Thie, D.C. in Touch for Health, this indicates what meridian is out of balance. We can then observe which chakra controls the meridian and which body needs balancing. When we correct the muscle imbalance, we also balance the chakra and Body to create a deeper pattern of ease.

And by the way: The purpose for all kundalini yoga kriyas is to balance this energetic flow.

LOCATION

Location is similar to Body Part, except that it indicates the paths where these meridians travel to the extremities. For example, if you have pain on the outside of the arm it could be one of three meridians, either large intestine/lung, glandular system, small intestine, triple warmer, or small intestine.

It is helpful to narrow down as much as possible exactly where the pain is. This will clue you in as to which meridian is malfunctioning which will lead you to the body or chakra which is out of harmony and this can lead to the deeper causal level of the dis-ease.

- Outside Leg: all Air signs
- Inside Leg: all Water signs
- Outside Arm: all Earth signs
- Inside Arm: all Fire signs

SENSE

The Organ and Sense columns are similar, in that they refer to areas in which an experience of dis-ease may be experienced.

SENSE/SENSE ORGAN

Is an indicator, which reveals the disharmony of a tattva, a chakra, or a meridian.

ORGAN

The Organ and Sense columns are similar, in that they refer to areas in which an expression of dis-ease may occur.

First Chakra	Spleen meridian	Stomach meridian	Earth Tattva	Taste
Second Chakra	Kidney meridian	Bladder meridian	Water Tattva	Hearing
Third Chakra	Liver meridian	Gallbladder meridian	Fire Tattva	Sight
Fourth Chakra	Large Intestine meridian	Lung meridian	Air Tattva	Smell / Touch
Fifth Chakra	Small Intestine meridian	Heart meridian	Ether Tattva	Speech
Sixth Chakra	Triple Warmer meridian	Pericardium meridian	Oversees first 5 chakras	ESP

NEGATIVE EMOTION

For example inflexible thinking would indicate a weak spleen/pancreas energy circuit. These indicators were obtained from Mishio Kushi back in the early seventies. By observing the emotions displayed or described, it could lead you to find out which of the 10 bodies needs to be balanced. See more under POSITIVE EMOTION.

TIME OF AGGRAVATION & ACTION

This column indicates both the time when the discomfort is experienced as well as the best time to do the intentional action. It indicates those hours in which the energies of the meridian system are most receptive to re-patterning by utilizing the healing influence of the light from the higher realms.

POSITIVE EMOTION

Charge	Meridian	Negative Emotion	Positive Emotion
Positive	Stomach	Exclusive	All Embracing
Negative	Spleen/ Pancreas	Inflexible	Flexible
Positive	Bladder	Pessimistic	Optimistic
Negative	Kidneys	Fearful/ Worried	Fearless
Positive	Gallbladder	Intolerance	Tolerance
Negative	Liver	Anger	Friendly
Positive	Lungs	No understanding	Understanding
Negative	Large Intestine	Unsteady	Steady
Positive	Heart	Coward	Brave
Negative	Small Intestine	Critical	Uplifting
Positive	Pericardium	Nervous	Calm
Negative	Triple Warmer	Emotional	Devotional

When someone creates the attitude of intolerance as a long-term stance in life, the gallbladder meridian will begin to spin in its opposite direction. The normal function of the gallbladder meridian is to disperse but when it spins in reverse, it will start to congest. To heal the underlying energetic pattern the person will need to address the emotional pattern of intolerance.

CELL SALT

Cell Salts are a profound way to smooth over the shortcomings in the foundational materials of the body. The tissues are very susceptible to imbalances because of their elemental makeup. This has as much to do with the elements in the Western sense as it does the Eastern. In other words, there are mineral deficiencies which supplemental cell salts help to correct. The way the researcher, Dr. Schuessler, who pioneered this field described the process is simple: salt is a crystal; crystals refracts light. What that means is that the patterns of light outside the body play a part in the functions within the body's energetic structure affecting its daily operations and especially in its chemical reactions.

1st CHAKRA

KALI MUR - Kali Muriaticum; Potassium Chloride
- White mucus, swollen glands.
- White or gray coated tongue, glandular swellings, discharge of white, thick mucus from nose or eyes.

CALC FLUOR - Calcarea Fluorica; Calcium Fluoride
- Poor tooth enamel.
- Cracks in palms of hands, lips.
- Hemorrhoids.
- Indigestion from rich food.

2nd CHAKRA

NAT PHOS - Natrum Phosphoricum; Sodium Phosphate
- Simple morning sickness; acid rising in throat.
- Headache on crown of head, eyelids glued together in morning.

- Grinding of teeth in sleep.
- Pain and sour risings from stomach after eating.

CALC SULPH - Calcarea Sulphurica; Calcium Sulphate
- Sores that heal poorly, herpes blisters.
- Pain in forehead, vertigo.
- Pimples on the face.

3rd CHAKRA

NAT MUR - Natrum Muriate; Sodium Chloride
- Dryness of body openings, clear thin mucus.
- Effects of excess overheating; itching of hair at nape of neck.
- Early stage of common colds with clear, running discharge.

FERRUM PHOS - Ferrum Phosphate; Ferrum Phosphate
- First stages of inflammation, redness, swelling, early fever.
- Congestive headache, earache, sore throat.
- Loss of voice from overuse.

4th CHAKRA

KALI PHOS - Kali Phosphoricum; Potassium Phosphate
- Mental/emotional symptoms predominate.
- Feel as if "I'm too tired to rest."
- Anxiety, brain fatigue, irritability, temper-tantrums, sleeplessness, dizziness.
- Nervous asthma.
- Easily bleeding gums.

NAT SULPH - Natrum Sulphuricum; Sodium Sulphate
- Green stools and other excess bile symptoms.
- Sensitive scalp.
- Greenish-gray or greenish-brown coating on tongue.
- Influenza.

5th CHAKRA

MAG PHOS - Magnesia Phosphorica; Magnesium Phosphate
- Muscle spasms, cramps and menstrual cramps, always better with heat.
- Hiccups.
- Trembling of hands.
- Teeth sensitive to cold.

KALI SULPH - Kali Sulphuricum; Potassium Sulphate
- Yellow mucus, later stages of illness.
- Congestion and cough worse in evening.
- Dandruff, yellow coated tongue, yellow crusts on eyelids
- Gas, poor digestion.

6th CHAKRA

SILICEA - Silica
- White pus forming conditions, boils - "homeopathic lancet".
- Stony-hard glands.
- Sty in eye area, tonsillitis, brittle nails.

CALC PHOS - Calcarea Phosphorica; Calcium Phosphate
- Post nasal drip.
- Upset stomach.
- Chronic cold feet.
- Poor dentition.

TASTE

Just as all the tattvas exist in composite form within the body, the ancient Indian art of Ayurveda teaches that every taste should be included in every meal. Just as with the elements, inclusion of these various tastes creates balance. For example, if you crave sweets, this would lead you in the chart to notice what organ would be affected and you would find the spleen/pancreas meridian. This could lead you to the causal factor to be the 1st chakra and 1st Body.

COLOR
Based on Chinese healing and not the yogic chakra colors.

Everything is made up of electromagnetic energy, which vibrates at different frequencies, which correspond to sound, light and color. We are drawn to the colors needed to create balance in our lives, the goal in all healing. Colors are frequency wavelengths that we connect with based on grid/matrix attraction and can be expressed in: clothing, accessories, colors in our homes, and even the foods we eat.

According to Chinese medicine by including the colors listed in the chart, through herbs and foods we can harmonize the function of the meridians/chakras/Bodies.

> **White:** cauliflower.
> **Yellow:** squash.
> **Red:** tomato.
> **Black:** black beans.
> **Transparent:** cucumber, orange, lime.

In addition, the color column refers to light as it is reflected through the various pigments. These can refer to food, as all meals should contain some of each color, and also to jewelry or colors painted on the walls at home. In each case, the way the light manifests itself helps facilitate healing and improve life.

AFFIRMATION

Sound is the most direct means into the psyche because it carries with it a charge that can be emotional and therefore deeply impactful. This notion actually gained some support from modern Physics, which has essentially verified the fact that all matter—your hand as well as the planet Neptune—is vibrating. That means everything gives off a sound, whether it can be heard or not. Those words and sounds that are both generated from and received by the psyche have actual, physical weight presence. Think about being in high school and someone was rude. When those words are taken in and cause a fear response, there can be a direct impact on the kidneys.

Emotions that become commotional are the blocks to personal growth because every person is subject to subconscious motivations. The long process envisioned by the ancient yogis was in essence, a patient re-patterning of these karmic impressions to engender new habits that achieve excellence and total fulfillment.

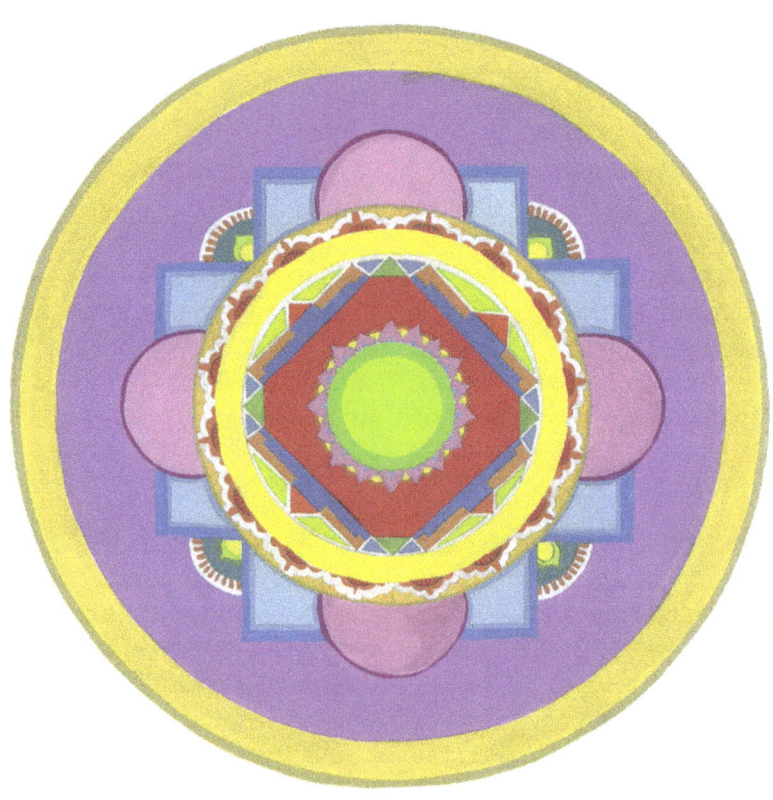

AFFIRMATIONS TO STRENGTHEN THE CHAKRAS

1ST CHAKRA	I AM CREATIVE, HUMBLE AND MY HEART RULES MY HEAD
2ND CHAKRA	I AM CONNECTED, OBEDIENT AND CONTAINED
3RD CHAKRA	I AM BLISS, THY WILL IS MY WILL, I SEE ALL AS EQUALS
4TH CHAKRA	I AM A YOGI, COMPASSIONATE, INTEGRATED, READY TO SERVE
5TH CHAKRA	I AM A TEACHER, BALANCED, I SACRIFICE FOR MY HIGHER SELF
6TH CHAKRA	I AM INTUITIVE, CONTROL MY PROJECTION AND PROTECTION, SEEK JUSTICE FOR ALL
7TH CHAKRA	I AM SELF CONTAINED, SECURE, FULL OF LOVE AND BENEVOLENCE

The first sutra in the Yoga Sutras by Rishi Patanjali's states:

Yoga is experienced in that mind which has ceased to identify itself with its vacillating waves of perception.

The reason we have affirmations in the guide is because four of the eight limbs of yoga have to do with the mind: pratyahar, dharana, dhiyana, Samadhi. This means that half of your practice needs to be dedicated to develop a mind, which has ceased to identify itself with its vacillating waves of perception.

The mind vibrates to one thousand thoughts per second, because of its connection to Chitta, the universal mind. It is made of the same stuff, which is ever moving, ever creating. The mind obviously cannot process all those thoughts to a harmonic neutral, so what happens with all those unprocessed thoughts? They end up with an electrical positive or negative charge in your subconscious. When the subconscious does not get cleared it starts to affect your life with nightmares, daydreams, and unfounded fears. In the same way, when a physical body gets filled with toxins it starts to produce pain, and when the mental body gets clogged up with toxins it also produces pain, dis-ease. One way to affect the mental field is to not dwell on those thoughts that cause you discomfort. When you are listening to a radio station and don't like the song, you can change stations. Apply this simple technique to your mind. When you are tuned into a station, which is broadcasting depression, sadness or overwhelm, change the channel. We suggest that you take the positive affirmation and use it consciously during asana practice, you can even write it on your mirror!

EXAMPLES OF POSITIVE AFFIRMATIONS

FIRST BODY
When I dwell in my True Identity (SAT NAM), all is perfect, whole and complete. I experience humility when I let my heart guide my head. I call on the wisdom within because I am one with the creativity of the Universe. Out of this creativity, come all the answers, all the solutions, all the healing, and all transformation. I trust this, I know that it is my true identity and whatever I need to know is revealed to me and whatever I need comes to me in the right time, space and sequence. In gratitude I bow to these qualities of creativity and humility.

SECOND BODY
When I dwell in my True Identity, all is perfect, whole and complete. I recognize that deep within me is the longing to belong. I obey this longing and connect deeply to the light of my soul.

THIRD BODY
When I dwell in my True Identity all is perfect, whole and complete. I see myself and all other beings in the Universe as absolutely equal, perfect, whole and complete. Like the rays of the sun I shine love and light on everyone.

FOURTH BODY
When I dwell in my True Identity all is perfect, whole and complete. Filled with compassion, I integrate all aspects of my experiences, and experience life as a yogi. I serve to resurrect others and myself with compassion.

FIFTH BODY
When I dwell in my True Identity all is perfect, whole and complete. I keep my body in an intricate balance. I sacrifice (make sacred), when I teach others to experience their own brilliance. With the great joy of being a teacher I choose to speak words, which guide others to have the experience of their Infinite nature. Each cell in my body has divine intelligence. I recognize my body as a good friend.

SIXTH BODY
When I dwell in my True Identity all is perfect, whole and complete. My intuition guides me in my ability to manifest my projection and it protects me every moment. I now dwell and live as the light of my soul.

SEVENTH BODY
When I dwell in my True Identity all is perfect, whole and complete. I feel self contained and deeply secure within my spiritual identity. My kindness throughout the day uplifts and elevates all beings and all situations.

EIGHTH BODY
When I dwell in my True Identity, all is perfect, whole and complete. I self initiate my creative talents and abilities to flow through me and express in deeply satisfying ways. I am filled with

courage, and energy. Each breath connects my finite self to my Infinite Self.

NINTH BODY
When I dwell in my true Identity, all is perfect, whole and complete. Deep at the center of my being there is an infinite well of calm. I now allow this calmness to flow to the surface ---it fills my heart, my body, my mind, my consciousness and my very being. The more calm I experience, the more I have to give because the supply is infinite. Mastery comes from paying attention to the subtleties and I express all the aspects of my life like a master.

TENTH BODY
When I dwell in my true Identity, al is perfect, whole and complete. I express the radiance and brilliance of the light of my soul. I act with nobility and royal courage in all of my actions. I express my courage, which is confirmed with every action I take. My radiant body shines like the masculine sun, providing light to all other 9 feminine bodies. I am the loving, living, joyous, brilliant expression of life.

ELEVENTH BODY
When I dwell in my true Identity all is perfect, whole and complete.

I am creative, connected to my higher self, blissful, a yogi, completely balanced, intuitive, self contained and courageous, I master and use my radiance unto Infinity to affect the change towards a brighter world with each breath.

NAAD YOGA
Connected through one sound current, the Naad, all manifestation has a vibration. In fact, philosophically speaking, a given frequency of vibration is what a being is. Everyone is pulsating at the rhythm of being human, and within that frequency, there are variations. Every column on the chart demands a certain degree of self-initiation, but none more so

than this one. Sacred sounds and mantras provide us with a codified, systematic use of sound for the purpose of decongesting clogged energy vessels, like the meridians and chakras. Re-orienting these vessels with new patterns, leads to the capacity to achieve your Purest Potential. This Naad sound was developed in accord with the concepts of ancient texts, which revealed that every sound possible from the human palate held a specific, universal meaning. In practicing mantra yoga, these sounds actually create the positive emotions associated with balanced chakras. The mantra sheet in the appendix describes mantras to balance the Chakras/Bodies.

TATTVA BALANCING

The Sikhs have five symbols, which they wear to balance the five tattvas; thereby minimizing reactivity to the outside world. They wear long hair to balance the ether tattva, a steel wrist bracelet, called a kara, to balance the air tattva, a small dagger called a kirpan, to balance the fire tattva and specially designed underwear, called ketcheras, to balance the water tattva. Finally, Sikhs put a small wooden comb in their rishi knot, the hair coiled on the crown chakra, to balance the earth tattva. We also know that yogis wear symbols like the earrings, a begging bowl, staff, conch and mala to balance the influence of the tattvas.

The most effective practice to balance all the tattvas is the Kirtan Kriya meditation. You can also do a yoga practice to generate a strong aura, as we now know that this magnetic force protects your identity by keeping all five tattvas together.

CHAPTER 7
APPLIED AWARENESS

There are many ways to apply the guide to your life. You will find some examples in this chapter. The biggest learning as you start out is:

**How to ask the right questions
so you can "read" where the imbalance is.**

It might not be the most obvious at first but as you investigate deeper, it will show up as the most consistent and relevant. In Australia, the aborigines look for "strings", indicators of imbalances, to show up in their meditation. When they find a string they hold on to it and follow it all the way back to it's beginning so they can shift the pattern of imbalance at its source. This is what the Guide provides for you, a place to locate your 'strings' so that you can hold on to them and follow them all the way back, and shift the patterns at a causal level. What we want to stay away from is the tendency to come up with a diagnosis of 'what ails you'. This is not the model we are promoting. Instead, recognize how the body, mind and spirit are interconnected and form this amazingly integrated structure, which continually seeks balance and homeostasis - harmony and ease.

The Guide presents all the places where you can receive a signal that something is out of balance. Use the Guide to locate the imbalance, and choose a practice to create balance. Continue investigating until the imbalance is corrected.

REAL LIFE APPLICATIONS FOR THE CHART

We once had a patient who had severe stomach problems with limited resources to make changes in his diet. There was also a great deal of skepticism around changing his food intake from the traditional diet he had grown up with. He had however, been raised with mantra yoga as a regular part of his daily life and was willing to recite a mantra 108 times per day.

He shared his results after reciting the mantra 108 times per day for 120 days; all pain had gone and the family now spoke about very positive and uplifting stories at the dinner table when previously arguments and topics which created fear and anger were talked about during meal times.

Mantra as a technique shifts the psyche through repetition of the harmonizing sound current. The specific mantra recreated the balance in the stomach meridian and made the patient aware of the patterns, which were causing the dis-ease.

A woman who had recently given birth came to the clinic. During the delivery, her liver had ruptured and there was internal bleeding to the point where she needed regular transfusions. She came in to see us wanting an alternative. This was a more serious problem than I was usually equipped to handle, but Dr. Schlesser's theories supplied me with the one recommendation I could make. Knowing her birthday, and that she was a Pisces, according to Dr. Schlesser's program, I suggested she take the appropriate Cell Salt for a Pisces, Ferrum Phosphate. Her western doctors were astounded at the suggestion. After bringing her into the hospital for an extended stay and flying in a special suit for her from NASA, they barred me from her room as they transfused more than 100 liters of blood over the course of a few days. Nothing seemed to work and they gave up. I was allowed to see her, at which point, I administered the Ferrum Phosphate and within seconds the hemorrhaging stopped completely.

The profound impact of the cell salts shows that these subtle mechanisms exist and to that end, begs the question: what is the nature of the relationship between people and light? The query is an ancient one and Dr. Schlesser ended up returning to this ancient approach in order to explain his findings. As the body takes in food to facilitate well-being, so does the ingestion of certain patterns of light facilitate healing for the subtle bodies. Because cell salt treatments work by reorienting the foundational materials in the body's chemical constitution to the light it's constantly absorbing, the cell salts provide an effective healing modality especially for meditators and yogis.

Once, a lady came to me with a sprained ankle. In interviewing her, she related a history of chronic sprains, always in her left ankle; never broken, but severely injured eight times over a five-year period. I was immediately clued into the Body manifesting a problem and intuited because of the association via the meridians of the ankles to the third chakra and, the possibility that the gall bladder organ might be imbalanced. I asked if there was any discomfort after a meal with fats (tattwa and chakra).

> Her answer was *"Yes, frequently."*
> I asked her: *"Do you have any pain near the scapula or headaches on the side of the head (gall bladder meridian)?"*
> *"Yes."*
> *"Do you like salt with your meals?"*
> *"Yes,"* she said, *"I always add some."*

I proceeded to order an ultrasound and we found gallstones. The symptoms in the Western assessment were arranged in a significant pattern according to the Eastern model of causality. In the end, the treatment was a realignment of habits. She changed her diet, adding artichoke tincture and a Cell Salt formula (Nat Mur 6x. Four tablets 4 times per day for 30 days). She practiced a yogic breathing technique to transform intolerance to tolerance. After some time, the stones were negligible and she was able to do a gall-bladder flush. At the last ultrasound, she had no stones present in her gall bladder, was symptom free and as to be expected, much happier. Furthermore, by making lifestyle changes to deal with an underlying cause of dis-ease, the patient self-initiated a series of reflections that led to the realization that she had been harboring intolerance toward her mother. Looking back, she saw each sprained ankle occurred after her mother came to visit her. In short, her healing was deepened on many physical and subtle levels.

The simplest way to conduct this kind of experiment is to begin changing habits regarding food. If there is a symptom or set of symptoms that correspond on the chart, adjust the diet to address the pattern of dis-ease. For example, if anger seems to be bubbling up out of nowhere and there is eyestrain and sore feet at the end of the day, add sour tasting and more green foods in your diet. Sour and green foods will add more harmonizing responses to the psyche and could lead to less and less anger reactions.

Now it's your turn:

There are many ways to do readings from the guide. Here are some ideas to get you started. The only agreement we need to make before you start to use the Guide is this..... You will ONLY use this information to create awareness for deeper healing and joy and remember that there is nothing broken.

Ask yourself which of the following 2 starting points gives you some information by revealing a "thread":
1. Find your horoscope sign on the chart and read its description, anything resonate? or
2. At what time do you experience discomfort? Does this correspond to any other symptoms on the chart? or
***If neither approach reveals your "string", try this one: How do you respond to pressure? Read on...

To find out where our opportunities for transformation are, Ram Das suggests that we spend a week with our family. What happens to you when you get under pressure? When we squeeze an orange, we get orange juice, when we squeeze a lemon we get lemon juice, when you get squeezed what comes out of you? Visiting your family might not pressure you, instead you feel pressure when you need to pay your bills, or when an appliance breaks down, when a friend does not call, or when someone cuts you off on the road. Reflect on your stress response and then circle the most prevalent emotion, which you express when under pressure:

Inflexible, pessimistic, exclusive, worry, fear, intolerance, anger, no understanding, unsteady, fear, critical, nervous, emotional

Look at the Negative Emotion column on the chart and follow the string this provides.

SOME OTHER WAYS TO READ THE CHART

Do a 5-minute pranayama: inhale left nostril, exhale right, inhale right and exhale left.
Check in with how your physical body has been feeling lately. Have you experienced any aches or pains? If so, where? Look this up on the chart and find out what intentional action you can apply to bring more balance in this area of discomfort.

Now that we have a way to regain balance and harmony with our Dharma, it's time to review a yogic method to share our Dharma with the world.

CHAPTER 8
PURUSHARTHA
For the Purpose of the Soul

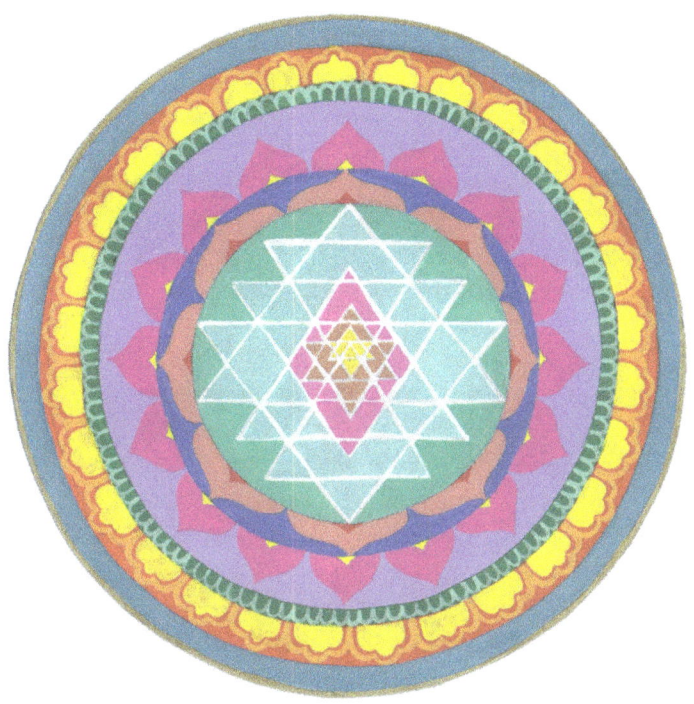

We all have something in common,
we breathe.
We vibrate and that vibration is the source of our life.
Life's magnetic field always surrounds us,
it is the psyche of individual existence,
which creates its magnetic field.
A human is a magnetic field, vibrating to its own nucleus.
You are the creative source and nucleus of the
whole vibratory effect in which you live.

Because we breathe, we are inherently creative beings. We create with our personal choices. The physical manifestation of our life is the outcome of our vibratory signature. With awareness of the ten bodies, we have learned to read both our vibratory effect and how to make course corrections. The process so far has been personal, yet the way to liberation is to take that personal experience and to share it with the world.

To do this as a yogi we suggest a brand new application of an age-old method for manifestation, which puts you at the center of the creative cycle. Purushartha is what the yogis identified as the cycles of creation, which are observable within you as well as in the world. We have found that it's the system, which attunes you to your vibratory nucleus, your Sat Nam, so that your actions can flow from an awareness of being.

The cycles of creation are virtuous, meaning they are based on universal principles and this was observable to the yogis who codified it and with some study they can become observable to us.

The yogis and mystics found that all energy manifests in a cyclical manner, and that these cycles manifest as the micro and macrocosm of life.

We will share a brief overview of how Purushartha can radically shift how you enter into your spiritual practice and the way you make your contribution in the world.

Purusha means – 'being' or 'soul'
Artha means 'ability' or 'for the purpose of'
Put together it means: 'for the purpose of the soul'

The Purusharthas are described extensively in the Mahabharata, the epic Indian poem contained in the Bhagavad Gita, and they are interwoven with yogic philosophy at the deepest levels. They have their roots in the Rig Veda, the most ancient and revered of Hindu scriptures. What the Rig Veda suggests is that the Purusharthas are the inherent values of the universe. The cosmos is considered a living being, and the four concerns of **Clarity (Moksha), Freedom (Kama), Stability**

(Dharma) and **Security (Artha)** belong to it. These are not just human concerns or psychological concepts, because when we engage with these concerns personally we have the potential to align the microcosm with the macrocosm.

The traditional utilization of the Purusharthas is to relate to them as aims or goals in life. With the Purest Potential application you will learn how to observe them personally, so you can more effectively influence the whole vibratory outcome in which you live.

We will now look at just a few aspects of the Purusharthas and begin the exploration of this approach. Of course, the applications are vast and this chapter will only touch the surface, just enough to observe how this could benefit you as a self-sensory being!

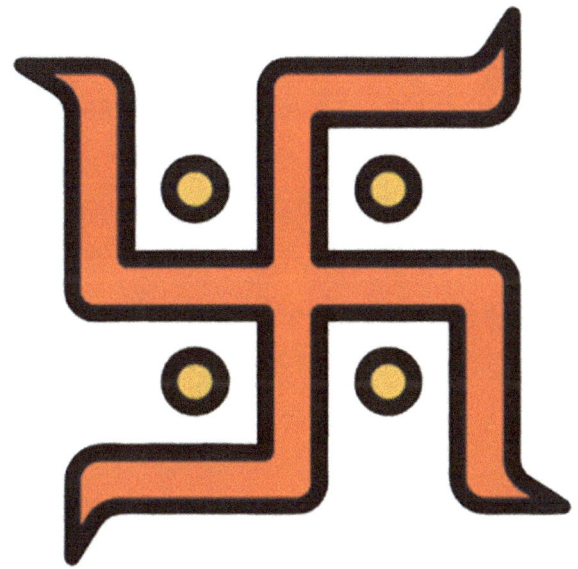

THE FOUR QUADRANTS

Each of us embodies one of the 4 purusharthas. Similar to astrology where you embody one of the 12 zodiac signs, in Purushartha, you embody one of the 4 quadrants. These quadrants present the fundamental ways in which people observe life and also how they make their contribution in the world. It is the lens through which we observe all of life. These four aspects of the manifestation wheel/cycle contain one of the four perspectives from which we each operate. Each person identifies with one aspect of the manifestation cycle. (We repeat this so often because in the beginning of this process many feel that they are all the quadrants!) When we are not clear about the quadrant from which we operate, we incorrectly assume that others have the same perspective as our own. When we are aware of these different concerns and perspectives, new possibilities become available for coordination of action and support. Cooperation and creativity replaces competition and confrontation.

QUALITIES FOR EACH QUADRANT

	MOKSHA	KAMA	DHARMA	ARTHA
Brings Forth:	Identity	Relationship	Value	Choice
Need For:	Control	Influence	Power	Authority
Language:	Declare	Promise	Request	Assert
Role:	Director	Facilitator	Builder	Analyzer
Actualizes:	Intention	Mood	Alliance	Assertion

We do operate in other quadrants, yet 'your' quadrant, will allow you to live in your purest potential. It is your "sweet" spot, so natural that you are usually the last one to even notice it. So, if you are confused after reading through this chapter about what your quadrant is, just ask a loved one which one they think you are!

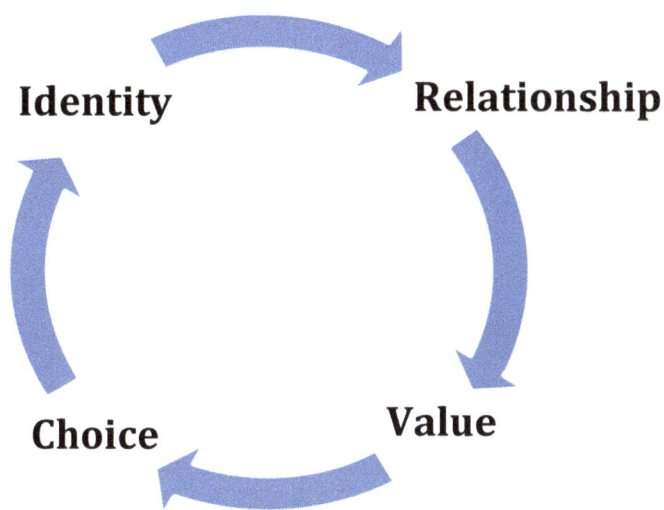

As you can see, each quadrant flows into the next, a beautiful harmonic circle with each aspect as important as the next. It represents a yogic model for a holistic and kinder experience for both our self and our world.

Please be mindful that you can use this system to become the expert at analyzing others and apply it as a fun "parlor game". However, the deeper application of the Purusharthas could be to express your brilliance, create conscious community in the process and make a positive change in the world!

Purusharta is always active because we are in constant relationship with nature's creative manifestation process. Our choice is to bring inner awareness to this process and flow with the cycles with intention and most importantly, TOGETHER!

MOKSHA – Certainty

Focused in realm of thought
Control
Marketing
Be
Intention
Yes= maybe, No=no

Natural qualities
Vision
Direction

Karmic qualities
Arrogant
Dictate
Manipulate

KAMA – Freedom

Focused in realm of action
Influence
Sales
View
Time
Yes=maybe, No= maybe

Natural qualities
Facilitate
Momentum

Karmic qualities
Impatience
Migrate
Sacrifice

DHARMA - Stability

Focused in realm of action
Power
Production
Do
Work
Yes=yes, No=no

Natural qualities
Results
Value

Karmic qualities
Frustration
Tolerate
Undermine

ARTHA - Security

Focused in realm of
thought
Authority
Administration
Review
Money
Yes=yes, no=maybe

Natural qualities
Evaluate
Integrity

Karmic qualities
Indifference
Hibernate
Betray

TWO CYCLES

The Purushartha wheel spins in 2 directions, and each direction has its unique application:

- Counterclockwise to contract into your inner still point
- Clockwise to expand into your contribution

The energy of the counterclockwise direction supports you to create a Bija, your inner still point from which you then manifest the mandala of your life.

The energy of the clockwise direction supports you to expand your offer externally out into the world. It brings forth your contribution.

Each of the cycles has a natural spin and because of free will the cycle can also be expressed in reverse. Each of us can consciously participate with these creative cycles by choosing to move with them in their natural expression, or not. All it requires as a self-sensory being, once again, is the ability to read your biology. The signs of how these cycles express are observable both within, as well as in the world. It is important to realize that once you find your quadrant there are 2 cycles you are a part of, both the inner and the outer cycles. These 2 cycles have a natural direction in which they move. When moving in the opposite direction there is stress, when moving in the natural direction there is ease.

	Clockwise	Counter-Clockwise
INTERNAL Your Sadhana	Dissipation	Focus
EXTERNAL Your Contribution	Expansion	Contraction

QUADRANTS AND CYCLES

Once clearly established in the natural contribution of your quadrant, you can observe the expression of the inner and outer cycles:

The natural spin when focusing within is counterclockwise

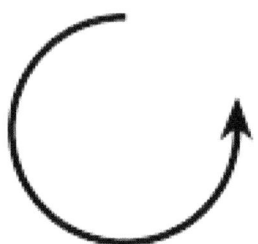

The natural spin when expanding into your contribution is clockwise

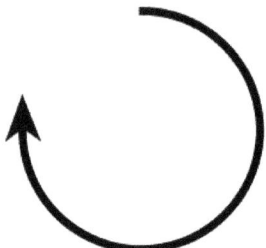

When energy is allowed its natural direction, the inner and outer expression of your life 'PULL' energy and manifest as peace and balance. This generates possibilities, the capacity for listening and elevated habits and choices.

When energy is applied in reverse; your inner and outer life become a constant "PUSH", a repeat of karmic patterns. And this "push" can be identified as stress, anxiety, blame, guilt, the same recurring emotional upsets and avoiding choice. This distress then becomes the basis for a scarcity or fear-based consciousness.

Let's see how these 2 cycles express for each of the quadrants.

MOKSHA

INTERNAL CYCLE - your Sadhana

- In the natural internal cycle the energy moves to the Artha concerns for accountability and security. When in this energetic flow it creates the capacity to observe results, which leads to more certainty.

- In the karmic internal cycle it moves to the Kama concern for freedom and engagement. When in this energetic flow a Moksha manipulates others emotions to achieve the outcome they want.

EXTERNAL CYCLE - your Contribution

- Moksha in the natural external cycle moves to the Kama concerns for freedom and engagement. In this natural expression of the cycle a Moksha engages a community by capturing the attention of others with their 'embodied' clarity!

- Moksha in the karmic external cycle moves to the Artha concerns for accountability and security, which expresses as manipulation as they turn their intention into an expectation and then become confused and manipulative to get others to give them clarity.

KAMA

INTERNAL CYCLE - your Sadhana

- Kama in the natural internal cycle focuses on the Moksha concerns for certainty and intention. This energetic flow creates certainty of their identity which expresses as the courage to make promises which connect others to the community.

- Kama in the karmic internal cycle move to the Dharma concerns for stability and power. When in this energetic flow they influence the outcome of interactions with their commotion to achieve the results they want.

EXTERNAL CYCLE - your Contribution

- Kama in the natural external cycle moves to the Dharma concerns for alliances and structure. When in this flow a Kama directs the powerful energy of feelings, with their courage and enthusiasm towards the alliances and structures, which connect others to the community.

- Kama in the karmic cycle moves to the Moksha concerns for clarity and certainty. When in this cycle they migrate and disengage to find their personal clarity. They get impatient, which they try to remedy by sacrificing themselves.

DHARMA

INTERNAL CYCLE - your Sadhana

- Dharma in the natural internal cycle moves to the Kama concerns for freedom and engagement, and this energetic flow allows Dharma to make fair requests, to bring greater value to the community.

- Dharma in the karmic cycle moves to the Artha concerns for authority and security and as the energy contracts they now use data to achieve personal stability and recognition. They only 'tolerate' (with much sighing) others as they push their version of work for personal safety.

EXTERNAL CYCLE - your Contribution

- Dharma in the natural external cycle moves to the Artha concerns for accountability and safety which allows them to feel stable and make requests which convert others to the community.

- Dharma in the karmic external cycle moves to the Kama concern of feelings which when a Dharma's efforts are not appreciated their response is to become frustrated which they try to remedy by undermining others.

ARTHA

INTERNAL CYCLE - your Sadhana

- Artha in the natural internal cycle moves to the Dharma concerns for structure and alliance, which creates the capacity for reflection.

- Artha in the karmic internal cycle moves to the Moksha concerns for clarity and intention. When in this karmic cycle they become ambivalent from analysis paralyses and hibernate.

EXTERNAL CYCLE - your Contribution

- In the natural external cycle an Artha moves to the Moksha concerns for clarity and intention. When in this energy flow an Artha gives constructive analysis, which brings the community into compliance to manifest the shared intention.

- Artha in the karmic external cycle moves to the Dharma concerns for alliances and safety. They seize authority in the community and then betray others to gain their own personal security.

THE AWARENESS JOURNEY

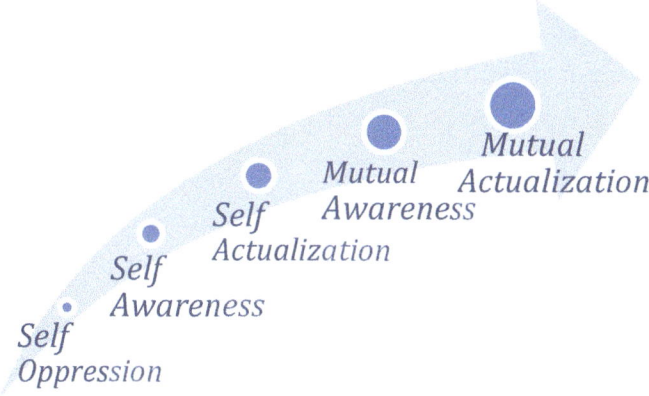

Self
Oppression

Self
Awareness

Self
Actualization

Mutual
Awareness

Mutual
Actualization

SELF OPPRESSION

We experience anxiety and fear in any of these quadrants when we strive to give ourselves what we are meant to give to the community. We self oppress when we are judgmental which can only produce agreement or disagreement and expect that this will change our future or support our intention.

We self oppress in each quadrant in these ways:
> <u>Moksha:</u>   When giving explanations.....anything after *"BECAUSE"*.
> <u>Kama:</u> When making empty promises.
> <u>Dharma:</u> When over-talking to create doubt and undermine the shared intention.
> <u>Artha:</u> When showing up a THE authority and make ungrounded assessments to get agreement or disagreement which polarizes the community.

With increased sensitivity to the Purushartha cycle, your sensations can inform you how to move into self-awareness.

SELF AWARENESS

Your quadrant is what you bring to the party and what you are accountable to deliver - it is your essential "truth". You don't need to be everything to everyone; you just need to deliver your natural talent. This is how we create conscious community, each person delivers their 'Sat Nam' with a shared intention for Purest Potential, a virtuous cycle. We practice Ten Body awareness and kundalini yoga to gain greater self-awareness of our essential nature, our Sat Nam.

Self Awareness for Each Quadrant:
> **Moksha:** Makes a declaration which provides for choice.
> **Kama:** Makes a promise which focuses time.
> **Dharma:** Make a request, which creates value.
> **Artha:** Makes a founded assessment, for reciprocal benefit.

SELF ACTUALIZATION

You can self actualize when you can be outside of your own concerns, which happens when your life is an expression of your quadrant's gift. When you are 100% accountable for standing in your clear offer and you speak from "BEING"

Moksha: Clarity and Intention.
Kama: Freedom and Engagement.
Dharma: Safety and Alliances.
Artha: Accountability and Security.

Self actualization can happen for each quadrant when these commitments are made:

Moksha: makes a declaration - a commitment to the future.
Kama: makes a promise - a commitment in the here and now.
Dharma: makes a request - a commitment to be satisfied when you do as I asked.
Artha: makes an assertion - a commitment to provide actual evidence.

MUTUAL AWARENESS

Happens when we as sovereign beings can listen to each other's listening. It happens when we commit to a learning community and give permission to others to call us out when we are off balance. Once you understand what your quadrant is and how the four quadrants operate together, it is important to remember that your tendency is to look at life from your quadrant's perspective, which will keep you in the state of Self Awareness. The opportunity to expand into mutual awareness happens when you can observe others not from your perspective but from theirs. When you can see the other quadrant's ways of seeing, and not fight the natural expression of the different quadrants because they are not like your own you are contributing to mutual awareness.

MUTUAL ACTUALIZATION

Is the natural outcome of the awareness journey. Mutual actualization has happened again and again in history. Take for example the Beatles: John is the Moksha, Paul the Kama, Ringo the Dharma and George the Artha.

> *"I am in you and you in me, mutual in divine love."*
> William Blake

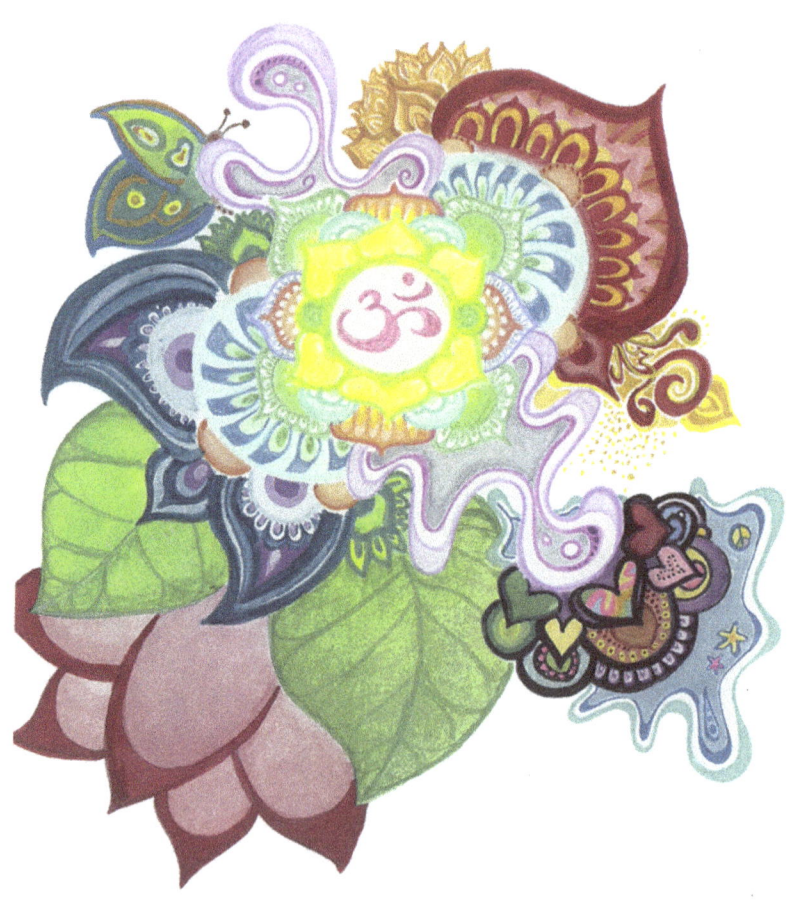

BALANCE - SHUNIA

Transformation can't be realized in a stable environment.

Balance is what is required to manifest your Purest Potential, and balance is what is lost when manifesting your Purest Potential. Your ko'an for the day!

In order to excel within the energy of these cycles you must confront all the habits, which keep you at your current level of growth. This opportunity is available when you loose your balance/dis-ease because change is what is required for transformation and for manifesting greater potential.

PRACTICE

When you observe yourself in breakdown, take a 'time out' to do this practice for greater balance. Do the practice until you sense your biology shift back to neutral. Once back to shunia, sit in stillness and meditate on your breath. Observe the guide and see new possibilities where there were none before.

<u>Moksha:</u> Sit in a meditative posture and lock the index fingers together in front of the heart center, pull the mudra and hold with Breath of Fire.

<u>Kama:</u> Same posture except lock the middle fingers together and keep a steady pressure with Breath of Fire.

<u>Dharma:</u> Same asana except lock the ring fingers together and keep a steady pressure with Breath of Fire.

<u>Artha:</u> Same asana except lock the pinky fingers together and keep a steady pull with Breath of Fire.
KEEP IT GOING and, remember this process has its own timing and we must develop our capacity for no immediate results......and to trust the process.

134

Some ways to practice the application of the Purusharthas:

1) **Be the observer of what is.**
   Observe the essence of nature, and how it manifests within and without. Kundalini yoga is the yoga of awareness, which is exactly what you need to observe the Purushartha cycle and deepen its application. So, do a daily kundalini yoga practice and keep a journal as you notice the expressions of Mokhsa, Kama, Dharma and Artha.

2) **Listen for other's listening.**
   Once you can observe the 4 quadrants the next move is to apply the meditative practice of shunia. Use your own stillness to listen for what others are listening for. They will tell you what their quadrant is, IF you can listen outside of your own concern (your own quadrant). The practice of Shunia gives you the capacity to listen outside of your own concern.

3) **Turn complaints into requests:**
   "What do you think you can do about that?"
   A complaint is an unspoken need. With awareness of the quadrants you can help others express the deeper need which is hidden in their complaint. It is amazing to observe how hard it is for most to discover what the deeper need is and to give themselves permission to actually ask for it! What is even more amazing is once you recognize their quadrant, the actual need will become so much easier to uncover.

4) **'You got to go before you know'**, get out in front of the Purushartha wave and stop getting ready to get ready!

   The process of transformation is inherently uncomfortable because it requires change and change is what most people avoid at all cost. Change requires new habits to support the new you. A goldfish kept in a fish bowl is used to swim in a tiny circle. When you place this

135

goldfish in an ocean guess what? The habit of swimming in a little tiny circle prevails even when the external environment has shifted. You, like this goldfish now have an entire ocean to swim in and if your habits are not upgraded they will keep you stuck in smallness. So take a risk and stop getting ready to get ready and create the new habits to venture out into that limitless ocean!

5) **Observe where the energy is being squandered** and observe that the actions, which got you to your current level of success can't create a breakthrough to the next level.

Life manifests in a circular pattern and we have seen some examples of this in the chakras, the wheel of time, and now the Purusharthas. When you observe that your current habits are keeping you from breaking through to the next level, then it's time to use the guide to set a new intention, which is aligned with a greater version of you! Some ways to deepen into this practice are to find a community committed to learning these principles, or to work with a Purushartha coach and learn how to apply these principles in your professional and personal life at www.purestpotential.com.

Don't worry if you didn't figure it all out! This is a vast area of study and it takes time to practice and actualize these principles. It's effective and might feel so 'right' to you because Purushartha confirms the natural expression of life, which is brilliant and prosperous. Never seen just one flower grow in a field, have you?

CHAPTER 9
COMMITMENT

Since you've made it this far, you've probably figured out that applying the information and methods will take commitment. At this point the overall intention for Purest Potential becomes imaginable, and some aspects of how to manifest it will apply directly to your life now, and some may never be especially relevant. At this time you have a complete picture of how and why your inner and outer environments feed the psyche information, and that <u>Self-Awareness</u> is the key to unlock the journey! By now you have a basic set of yogic tools for realistically implementing practices into your life to reveal more of your personal truth and to move forward with awareness in the process of Self - realization.

Commitment is what is required for this process to continue and for it to be sustainable in this polarized world full of distractions. Commitment is defined in the dictionary as: to make a pledge or a promise. Imagine you have a big clump of clay with a certain amount of time to create your masterpiece. The clay needs to be shaped and reshaped each day as your vision for what your masterpiece is gets more refined. Your capacity to commit to the daily "shaping" process is what makes the difference between wishful thinking and the brilliance of Self-actualization.

We will consider the topic of commitment by going through the 4 moves of the external Purushartha cycle, so that the energy can build on itself by following the natural expression of growth and expansion. Observe how the 4 quadrants have infinite ways to express. In our consideration for commitment it could look like this:

MOKSHA	WHY
KAMA	HOW
DHARMA	WHAT
ARTHA	COMMIT

Commitment is what happens in the Artha quadrant after each of the other quadrant's concerns has been managed to completion.

Let your powerful 'why' inform your choices and initiate the manifestation cycle.

Unless there is a clear why, the course of life will disorient and confuse you with all kinds of new and shiny objects to divert your attention. Our discussion in the Moksha quadrant is about your 'why'. Why do you want to commit to your own potential? Why do you want to spend your time and energy applying these practices? Is this reason powerful enough to keep you on course when the distractions of life show up as they will, and as they must?

In Tibet when a new student comes to the monastery the master will sometimes instruct the student to remain at the gate. Since this is not the West, this particular student knows not to ask, "For how long," or another favorite, "Why?" This student knows that the master is testing him to see if he has a clear intention, a clear why, to overcome his self- imposed limitations and fears. A student could sit outside in the rain and snow for awhile, until the master notices that the student is committed to his self-mastery.

Life is the process that brings the snow and rain to see if we can sit it through to the other side. How does that work? And how to stay on track? With a deep commitment you can recognize the moments when a decision on how to move forward is needed. We have all experienced the prevalent opportunity for standing in our power of choice; whether we have been able to commit to it or not, is the consequence of having or not having a clear why.

I went through a scary time in my marriage where I was squandering the energy and not able to create a breakthrough. After the first seven years of marriage I was swimming in my old familiar fishbowl of blame and pain and the energy kept building to give me the opportunity to create a breakthrough. I hit that place where he just couldn't do anything right, he became an obstacle between me, and the refrigerator and even between myself and my fulfillment. If it weren't for him, I figured, my life would just be so much easier, happier and more exciting. So one night, after yet another big drama played itself out, I ran away. This was my favorite way to respond to the pressure of having to face my fears. This time, however, I did not drive for hours in my car. Instead, I went and meditated in a pasture with a bunch of horses. As I sat in that circle of very curious horses, I observed that I had a back door —a door I could walk through when any part of my life got too hard or too scary. My opportunity at that moment of new awareness was to upgrade my why. My why was not to figure out who had been "right" in the fight. I had the choice to swim around in my karmic fishbowl or transform that energy and align my marriage with a new why. My why changed from 'he had to make me happy' to 'marriage is my path to self realization'. With that, I could commit to close the back door. Marriage did not necessarily get easier, it just became possible. From that new why, I could create a breakthrough to the next level.

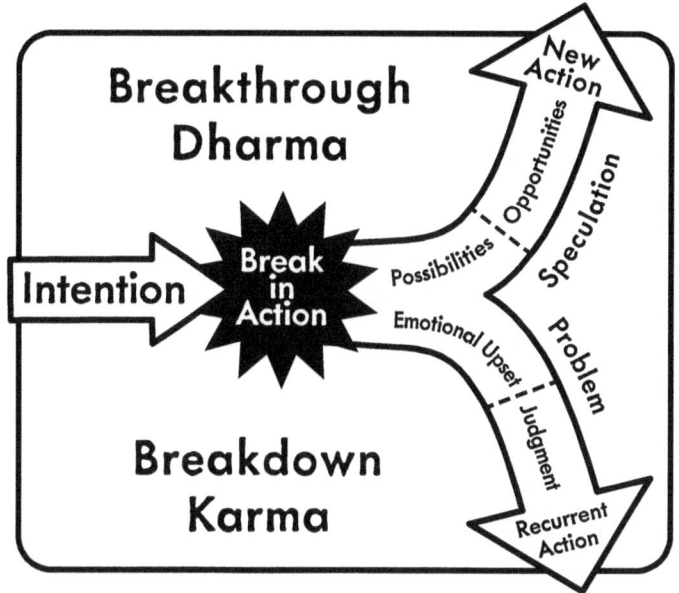

This image represents the Karma to Dharma or breakdown to breakthrough model. Know that there is not just one break in the action and that it is actually an ongoing process, one that asks us to level up typically just when we thought we had it all figured out! The place of breakdown offers 2 opportunities:

1) To do what you have done before, recycle your karmic story and stay in that breakdown

or

2) Stop and observe new possibilities and opportunities to create a new way forward

It's clear intention that creates breakdowns as it produces the possibility for transformation. It's clear intention that also creates the breakthrough, as it produces new choices. In other words always look to intention to initiate the manifestation cycle.

PRACTICE

At the end of the following practice we invite you to write down your declaration and initiate the Purushartha cycle for the sake of committing to your brilliance.

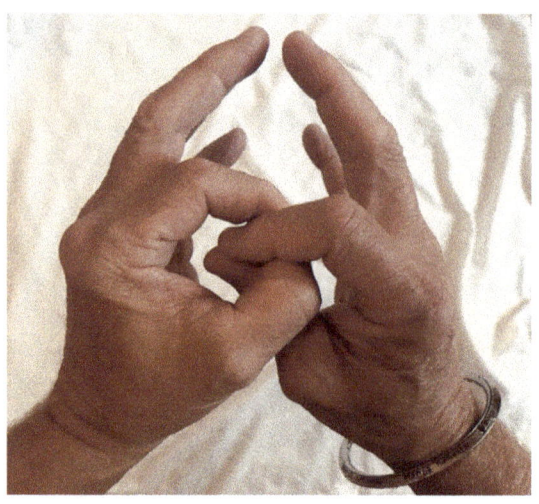

Sit in easy pose, hands in gyan mudra. Tips of the index fingers touch the tips of the thumbs and then interlock these two circles. Hold this mudra at the heart chakra in a relaxed way. Eyes look down at the mudra and keep the eyes fixed. Hold with relaxed breath for **3 minutes.**

Close the eyes and look at the 7th chakra, the 10th gate. Shoot your awareness out into Infinity, beyond and beyond, beyond space and time and observe your life from this vantage point. Let the body go. Be still and observe, allow a new reason to commit to your potential to reveal itself from this higher vantage point. Continue for **8 minutes.**

I commit to my brilliance, my purest potential because:
Write your (short) why at the top of the star

HOW

Engage with ONLY that which matters:

The way we move our intention forward is with the energy generated by sensations and emotions, the kama's forté! Once you declare your why, the Kama phase is how you actually will engage with it. Looking back at the breakdown>>breakthrough model, we can see that there are two distinct 'hows'. We can either engage with our karmic story or make the choice to manifest our dharma. Sensations and emotions illuminate this choice. Each choice will feel very different, one is familiar and the other requires risk and could feel a bit scary. When you engage with your karmic story, your choices perpetuate very familiar pain, adrenaline rushes, fear, anger, blame, and entangle you with deep attachments to being the best, the smartest, the fastest, the prettiest, youngest, wisest, calmest, etc. When you engage, instead, with your newly declared intention it requires courage! (another Kama forté).

When the Kama quadrant is not aligned with a clear 'why', your self-realization journey could express as "spiritual window-shopping." A lot of people take one thing from one tradition and another from the next, because it all feels so fun and enticing. This is fine while you are searching, but it is important to clarify your commitment sooner or later. In this commitment process you will recognize that you have a choice to be: "a mile wide and an inch deep or an inch wide and a mile deep". Being a mile wide expends a lot of time and diffuses your energy.

Trust yourself and the feedback your conscious engagement with the process to liberate restrictive patterns brings. At this point in the Purushartha cycle, you transform the intention for commitment into: every day courage!

PRACTICE
Pran Japa

*"To know all life, to go beyond time and space
to know past, present and see the future"*

Sit in easy pose with hands in Gyan mudra on the knees. Lift your weight up off buttocks, and sit very lightly. Feel you are pulling yourself up in the air and become very light.

Keep stretching the lower spine up, eyes are closed.

Inhale completely filling the lower, mid and then upper lungs. Pull body weight up and lift this energy into the head, let it completely fill the brain.

Exhale hold air in chest and release breath from the navel only, and let the body weight slowly flow outward with the breath and mentally chant 'Wahe Guru" 16 times.

Continue for **7 to 11 minutes.** At the completion, observe how to move your intention forward in the kama quadrant.

Example:

COMMIT   CALM

Your Turn:
- Write your *commit* on the left side of the star.
- Write your *'why'* on top of the star.
- Write your *'how'* on the right side of the star.

PUREST POTENTIAL

WHAT
Do that which brings greater value.

Once you are clear about why you want to commit and can engage with only with what matters, we bring the intention down to earth in the Dharma quadrant. The first two quadrants of Purushartha are similar to the offensive aspect of a team, and the move to the next two quadrants provides the defensive aspects for the game.

We secure the intention and make it real with our daily actions and the company we keep. The Dharma quadrant is one of power because your potency will shift from an inch deep and a mile wide to a mile deep and an inch wide. Purushartha is not about doing everything for everyone or doing the next new thing; it's about manifesting your intention. A Dharma will never do things on just faith, they would be the ones to ask: "What are you going to do to get that concrete result?" In this phase you focus your daily habits and actions to generate a specific and committed result. Now that is a real expression of power!

There are powerful yogic reasons why committed daily actions are so important. Healthy habits insure the proper functioning of each organ, creating a more powerful electric pulse at the end of each meridian. This in turn, demands that the energy of the nadis at each chakra is balanced according to the increased voltage. A more powerful magnetic field provides more stability to the chakra system. Turning up the power with committed daily actions creates stasis in the chakra, which allows the spin of each vortex to be less like a whirlpool and more like a pair of turbines spinning, side-by side in opposite directions. The effect of this motion is what draws the Kundalini upward through the sushumana. When this vital substance passes the energy field, the Body, of each chakra it produces a side effect, what the ancient yogis called "ras," literally meaning "juice" or "nectar." At this point, not only is each organ healthy and every passageway clear, all chakras and Bodies support the brilliance of the soul's light.

Another Dharma aspect which stabilizes the intention is through the association with what is known as a sangat. A sangat is made up of people that are not necessarily friends or family, but instead are other seekers, those who hold each other up to their higher values and who will not shy away from doing so because of societal norms and conventions. The process of transformation produces breakdowns and a community committed to learning is what anchors this process.

Example of the Purushartha Cycle:

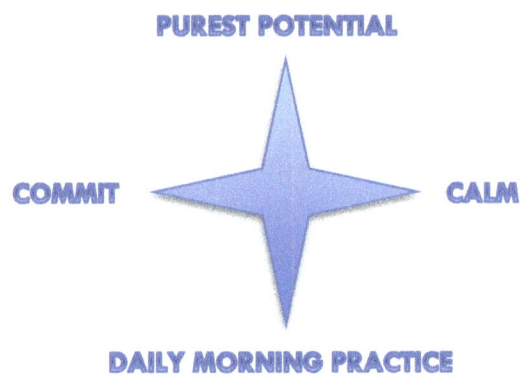

PUREST POTENTIAL

COMMIT — **CALM**

DAILY MORNING PRACTICE

Your Turn:
Write 'commit' on the left of the star, your WHY at the top, your HOW on the right, and your WHAT at the bottom.

COMMIT

Your capacity to commit in the Artha phase of the Purushartha cycle becomes possible once you have:
- a clear why,
- an exciting how and
- a valuable what.

Commitment is what continues to move the energy in an expansive direction. This sounds easier than it actually is, because our undisciplined default tendency in the Artha aspect of the cycle is to find what is wrong, focus on that and use it as evidence for 'why not'. This phase is where we commit to stay the course, it is where we choose to use data to support the intention and avoid getting stuck in 'analysis paralysis'.

In spiritual texts the path of the seeker is often described to be finer then the breadth of a hair. I once asked my brother in law, who is a professor of Physics, why the thread in my sewing case is always tangled, and why the garden hose always manages to get itself tangled up as well. He told me something very revealing, "There are endless opportunities to get something wrong and there is only one way to get it right". This realization that the odds of finding peace and harmony are slightly against us, is actually the reason why yogis and mystics advice us to commit to our discipline every day and, in a perfect world, with every breath. We commit to generate forward movement, which creates more prana to unwind the polarities (karma) and dwell in shunia.

Complete your Purushartha star once again!

Commitment is what keeps the process of transformation moving in the direction for continued growth. The expression of the 10 Bodies give feedback as to your level of commitment as well!

BODY	WITHOUT COMMITMENT	WITH COMMITMENT
1	Dull	Creative
2	Conspiracy us and them theories	Connected
3	Unmotivated	Bliss
4	Reactive	Resurrection
5	Selfish	Balanced
6	Spaced out, unfocused	Intuitive
7	Insecure	Self contained
8	Anxious	Courageous
9	Restless	Calm
10	Ineffective	Radiant
11	Confused	Mastery

CHAPTER 10
SELF-INITIATION INTO BRILLIANCE

For the times, they are a' changing. They will and they must because expansion is the essence of our universe and consequently of us. The tendency is to react to this process of continuous transformation by taking it all personally. The opportunity however is to observe this phenomenon for what it is, an expression of the nature of life. The process of transformation is impersonal yet requires our personal participation. So how do we dance successfully between the impersonal and personal? By knowing yourself! The 10 bodies provide constant feedback in this dance of continuous expansion. We can align with the profound energy of our subtle bodies when we enjoy a yogic lifestyle focused on deep listening, self - initiation and seva. During times of great transformation, it can feel like living in a foreign land as old familiar language and customs don't work any longer. Consequently, rather than try to mend what is outdated, it is a time to initiate change.

By now, it is clear that the Purest Potential methods give you the capacity to self initiate and ride this wave of transformation. The disciplines for greater Self awareness: yoga, meditation, the ten Bodies, and Purshartha, once learned, can be applied by you directly with no need for an intermediary. When you learn how to be the observer of what is, you can then choose your personal practice for transformation. There are two ways to grow and change, it is either through
>   time and space **or**
>   through the heat, the tapasia, of a personal practice.

Time and space are very effective teachers, whatever we need to learn just keeps showing up, with different faces in different places, and there is that same lesson again. When you self initiate a personal practice it puts you in front of this wave, so that you can literally ride the energy rather then be dragged by it.

At Purest Potential we have a fun way to remember the essence of the practice to self-initiate. We call this: assontheline. Our coach when explaining the Purushartha process drew this "universal symbol" on the board.

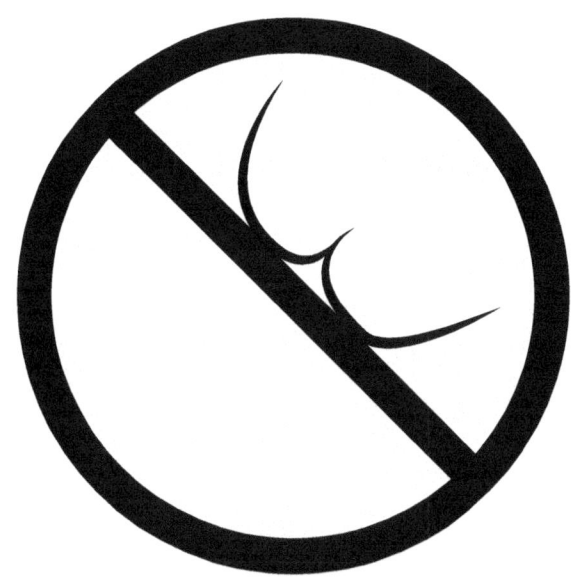

assontheLine

Then asked us what it was. After pondering many universal truths and not figuring it out, he shared the answer.....

Ass on the line.

Oh my, this very personal reference is not what we expected. What we expected was some universal ambiguous truth, which we could contemplate and pontificate over. Assontheline is the opposite of ambiguous, it is very up close and personal.

We've heard it said that angels pray for a human incarnation, because transformation can only happen in-body. We have an amazing opportunity to affect the macrocosm when we choose to self-initiate (assontheline) positive change.

There is a beautiful allegory in the Hindu tradition, which goes like this:

Lord Indra has a net which spans over all this universe and:
- at each juncture there lies a jewel;
- each jewel reflects all the other jewels in this cosmic matrix.
- Every jewel represents an individual life form, atom, cell or unit of consciousness.
- Each jewel in turn, is intrinsically and intimately connected to all the others;
- Thus, a change in one gem is reflected in all the others.

As you self initiate your healing and bring more awareness to your life, you automatically affect all other lives. Let your seva, your service, be to do a personal practice for positive global change. Not by creating more to do lists, but from greater intention and engagement.

> The wind is always blowing
> all you have to do is raise your sail!

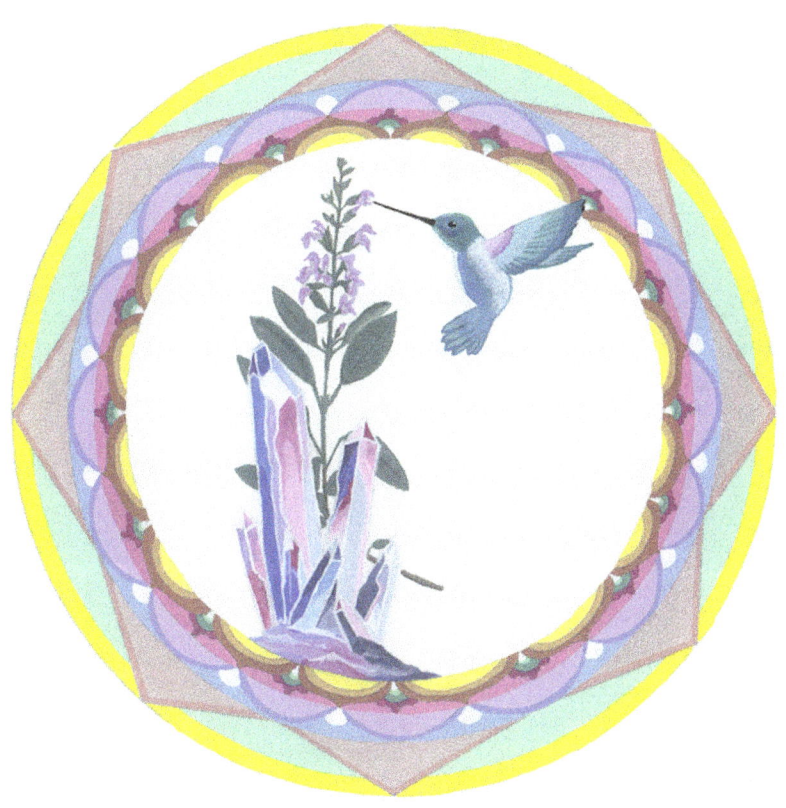

PRACTICE

Intuition is the principle for you Identity

Sit in easy pose. Lock fingers at heart chakra with index finger pointing up and thumbs crossed.

Eyes closed and mentally look at the horizon, straight (for stability)

After **3 minutes** begin to whisper powerfully: 'SA, TA, NA, MA' After **9 minutes** inhale, hold the breath and concentrate on the spine from the bottom to the top. Then relax and observe: the wind is always blowing all I have to do is to raise my sail.

I self initiate (assontheline) when I:
- Select practices based on the guide and my numerology.
- Eat food which supports my health.
- Practice yoga and meditation intentionally.
- Am aware of the numerology for each day.
- Review my day before I go to sleep.
- Declare my intention at the beginning of each day.
- Engage only with what matters.
- Produce that which brings greater value.
- Collaborate with others in the Purushartha way.

Time for ....assontheline. Write it down how you will self initiate your life!

Congratulations, you read the whole book. Each one of us affects the totality of our shared experience. May you experience the excellence of a fulfilled life and remember that your birthright is happiness. Thank you for being part of a new story where each person can:

- Declare their Purest Potential
- Transform emotions, generated by samskaras and karmic patterns, to devotion
- Practice their dharma
- And BE BRILLIANT already!

So much love and light and have fun with the practices on the next pages.

Stay as close as you can to your own experience

You are the alpha and the omega

**Breathe deep and tune in,
because all you have to do is
Be You.**

**May all beings be happy,
May all beings be at peace,**

Sat Nam

KUNDALINI YOGA KRIYAS

Start each Kriya or Meditation by tuning in with the
Mangala Charan Mantra explained on page 220

End your practice with the sunshine song
found on page 227

1st BODY
Kundalini Yoga Kriya
Heart Over Head - Align with your Soul

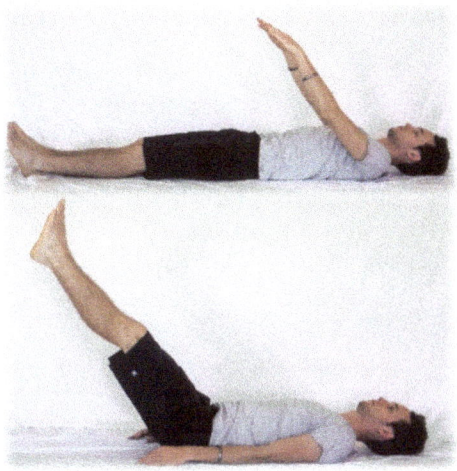

1) Lie on back, inhale and raise arms to 60°, and hold for a few seconds. Exhale bring arms down.

On next inhale raise legs 60 degrees, hold for a few seconds. Exhale lower legs down.

Continue alternating arm and leg lifts - **3 minutes.**

2) Lie on back, raise legs 90 degrees and hold for **1 minute** with long deep breathing.

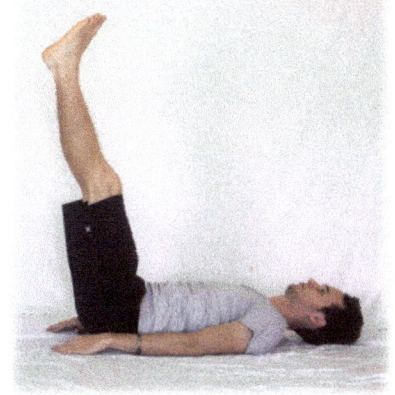

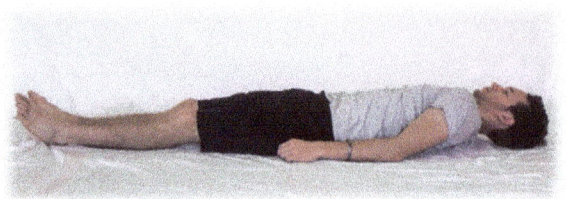

3) Lie on back, legs on ground. Put the heels together and press the toes forward, inhale and hold for **30 seconds** then relax on the back for **30 seconds.**

4) Lie on back, lift one shoulder up to the sky and then drop back to the ground, then lift the opposite shoulder. Continue to lift alternate shoulders off the ground for **1 minute.**

5) Lie on back and bring left knee to chest, raise the right leg to 12 inches and swing raised leg in a 180° arc from the hip for **1 minute**.

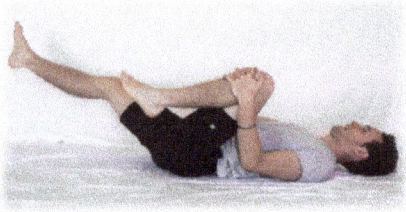

Switch legs and repeat this exercise with the other leg for **1 minute.** Repeat three times for **total of 6 minutes**.

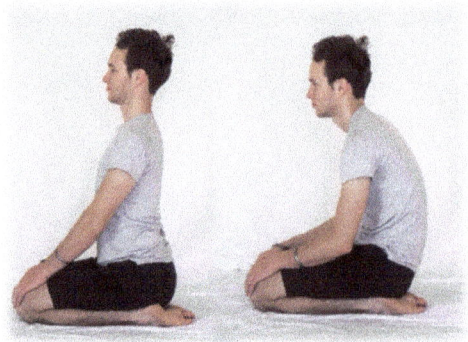

6) Sit in rock pose and do spine flex, hands rest on thighs for **2 minutes.** Fast!

Inhale flex the spine forward, exhale flex the spine back. The head stays level and only the lower spine moves.

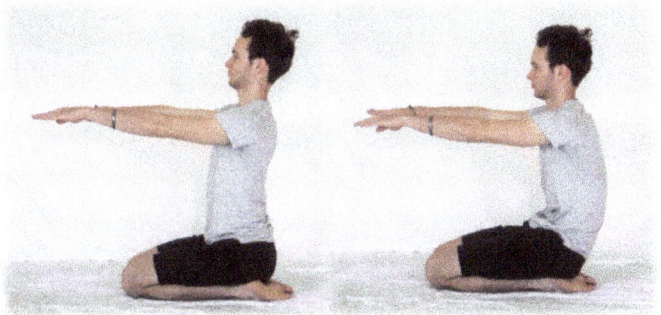

7) Continue spine flex in rock pose with the arms straight out in front with palms down for **2 more minutes**.

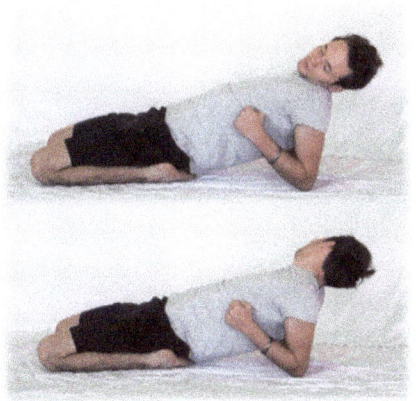

8) In rock pose, lean back on the elbows and begin to roll the neck for **1 minute** in one direction and then switch and roll in the other direction for
1 minute.

9) Repeat Exercise #4, lie on back lift alternate shoulders this time with Breath of Fire for **3 minutes.**

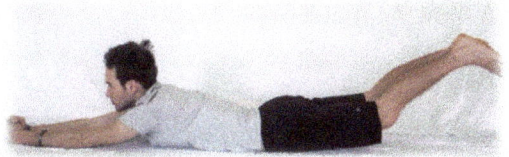

10) Lie on stomach with arms extended out in front and hands in Venus lock, raise the head and legs (**not** arms) 6 inches with Breath of Fire for **1 minute.**

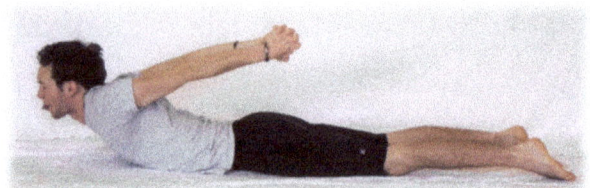

11) Lie on stomach with hands on the lower back in Venus lock. Raise the head and arms (<u>not</u> legs) as high as you can, curl your tongue and do Breath of Fire for **1 minute** through the curled tongue.

12) Dynamic Cobra pose. Lift up in cobra pose and chant "HUM," then exhale and when chin almost touches the ground chant "HUM". Keep elbows close to sides. Move up and down chanting for **3 minutes.**

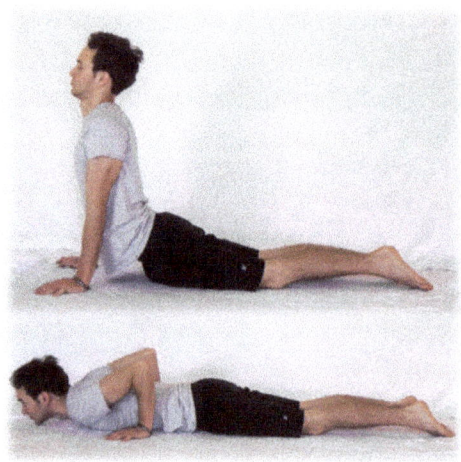

13) Shavasana **11 minutes.**

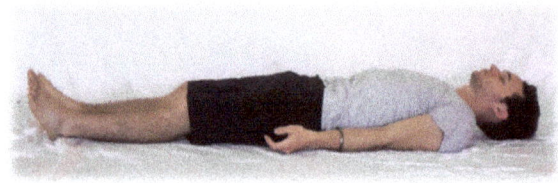

1st BODY
Kundalini Yoga Meditation
Heart Over Head – Meditation to Open the Channels

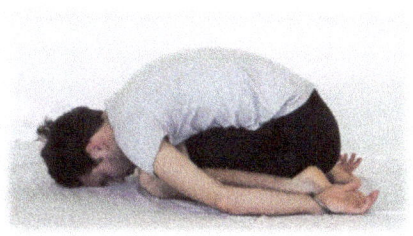

PART 1
Celibate pose. Sit on the heels and then sit in between heels in celibate pose. Place forehead on the ground.

Alternate position: Sit on heels and interlace hands behind neck, elbows point to sides.

Inhale and exhale apply Mulbandh. Hold for 2 mental repetitions of 'SA TA NA MA'

Release Mulbandh. Continue for **15 minutes.**

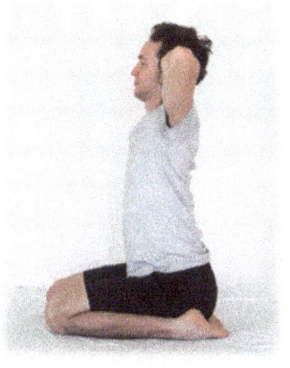

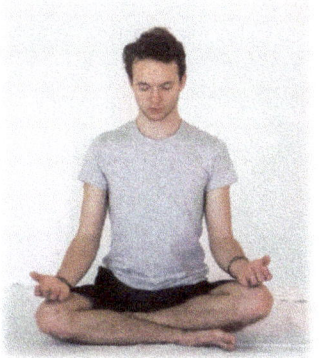

PART 2
Sit in easy pose with Long Deep Breathing for **11 minutes.**

PART 3
Lie on back and listen to mantra: 'EK ONG KAR, SAT GUR PRASAD, SAT GUR PRASAD, EK ONG KAR'

2nd BODY
Kundalini Yoga Kriya
Longing to Belong - Connect with your Soul

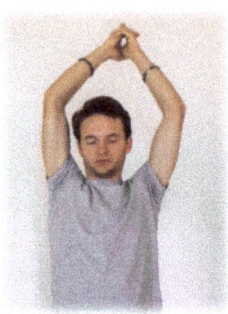

1a) Stand with arms raised and clasped above head, index fingers point upward.

With a very small motion: inhale as you lean forward, exhale as you lean back. **Continue for 1-3 minutes.**

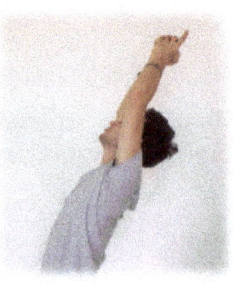

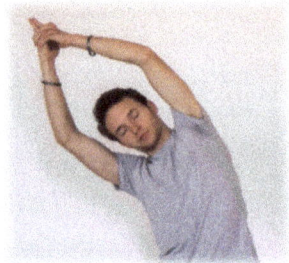

1b) Stand in same posture and lean to the right as far as you can. Press outside of left foot into the ground and lengthen the whole left side of the body. Hold with long deep breath for **1½ minutes.**

1c) Same posture and lean to the left as far as you can for **1½ minutes**. Press outside of right foot into the ground and lengthen the whole right side of the body.

1d) Same posture move arms in large circles from left to right for **1 ½ minutes** then switch direction and move from right to left for **1 ½ minutes.** Draw a large circle with your index fingers in the sky.

2) Stand with legs shoulder width apart and raise arms up to 60°, palms face forward. Inhale then very slowly exhale and squat down half way, **continue 1½ minutes.**

Put heels together and continue for another **1½ minutes**

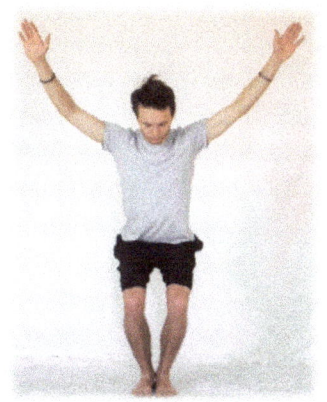

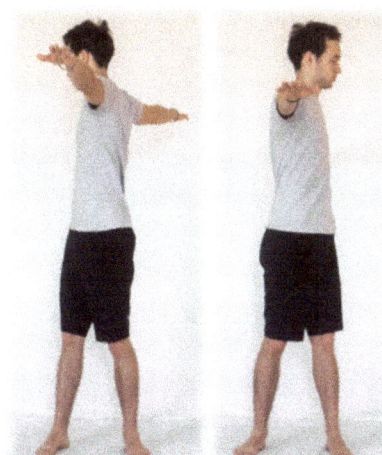

3) Stand with arms out to the side, palms face down, parallel to ground. Inhale center, exhale twist to the left, inhale center, exhale twist to the right.

Continue 3 minutes.

4) Come into triangle or downward dog. Lift left leg to 60 degrees and hold with Long deep Breathing. **1½ minutes**

Lift right leg to 60 degrees with long deep breathing. **1½ minutes.**

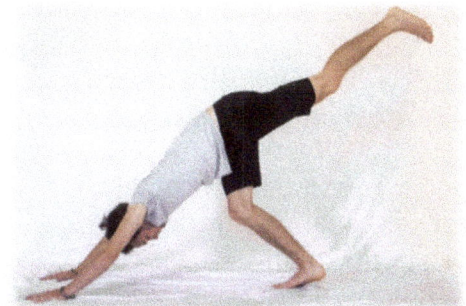

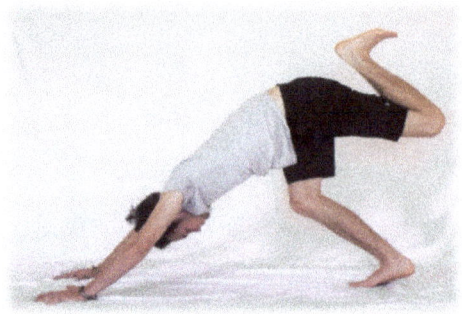

Lift left leg and kick buttocks with left heel. **1½ minutes.**

Lift right leg and kick buttocks with right heel. **1½ minutes.**

5) On all fours with the spine in a neutral position. Hold posture, keep knees on ground and kick buttocks with alternate heels, exhale when the heel strikes the buttock. **Continue for 3 minutes.**

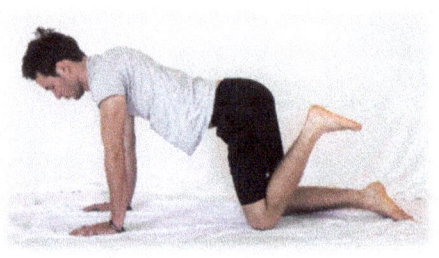

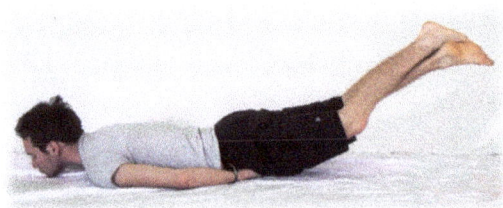

Continue for 2 minutes.

6) Locust pose, chin on ground, fists on either side of pubic bone, cross legs and lift legs up with Breath of Fire.

7) Bow pose with Breath of Fire. **Hold for 1½ minutes.**

In Bow pose begin dynamic rocking motion inhale up, exhale down.

Continue 1½ minutes.

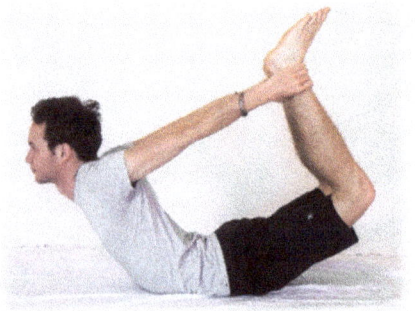

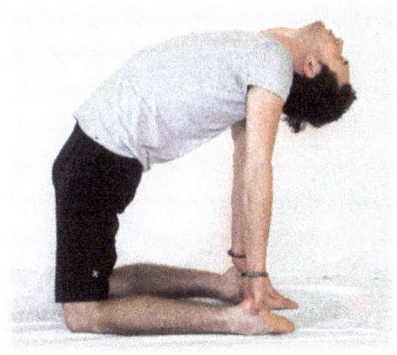

8) Camel pose. On heels, come up on knees, press hips forward and lean back, hold ankles, drop head back with Breath of Fire. **3 minutes.**

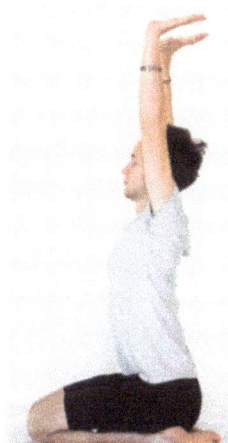

9) Sit on heels. Arms above the head, palms flat as if holding a tray, fingers point toward the back.

Inhale up and exhale bow with palms flat on ground in front. **Continue for 11 minutes.**

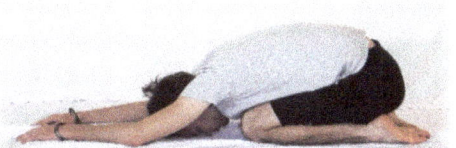

10) Shavasana.

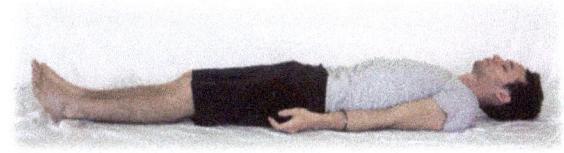

166

2nd BODY
Kundalini Yoga Meditation
Longing to Belong - Connect with your Soul

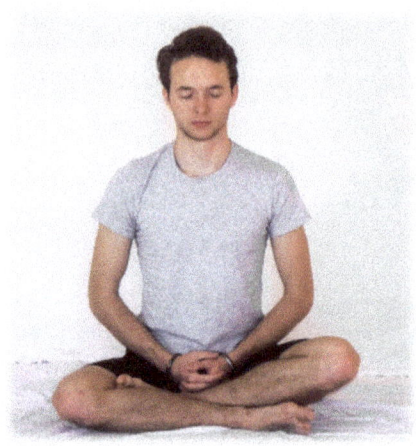

Sit in Easy pose with hands in Venus lock resting in the lap.

4 Part Meditation

- Apply Mulbhand and chant 'WAHE GURU',
- Release Mulbhand chant 'SAT NAM' and
- Apply both Mulbhand and Diaphragm locks and Chant 'HARI HARI',
- Release bandhas and chant 'RAM RAM'

Continue for 11 – 31 minutes.

3rd BODY
Kundalini Yoga Kriya

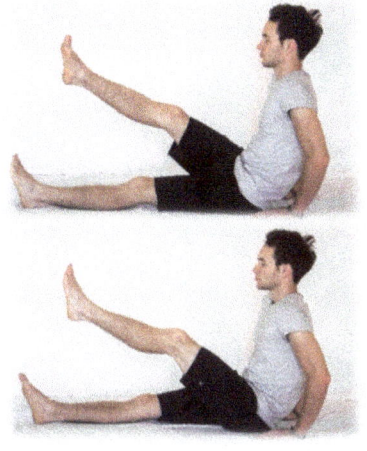

1) Sit with legs out in front. Lean back with neck lock engaged. Arms by sides, hands next to hips, shoulders relaxed, heart open. Inhale lift left leg up to 60 degrees, exhale down, inhale lift right leg up to 60 degrees exhale down. **3 minutes.**

2) Same posture and lift both legs up to 60 degrees. Lift arms parallel to ground, palms down. Breath of Fire. **1 minute.**

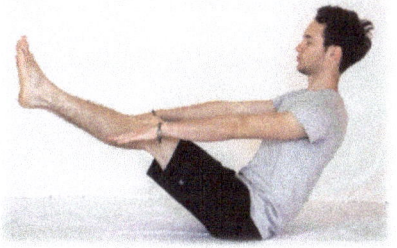

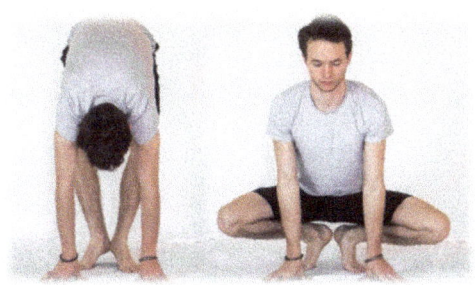

3) Frog pose with heels off the ground. Inhale straighten legs, exhale squat down. Continue for **1 - 3 minutes**

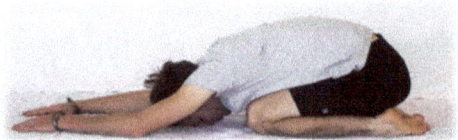

4) Guru Pranam. On heels, fo rehead on ground arms stretched out in front, palms down. Inhale, exhale apply vigorous Mulbhand or root lock, and release on exhale, continue for **3 minutes.**

5) Lie on back with hands by hips, palms up. Inhale raise both legs to 90°, exhale legs down with a long and slow breath. **1 - 3 minutes.**

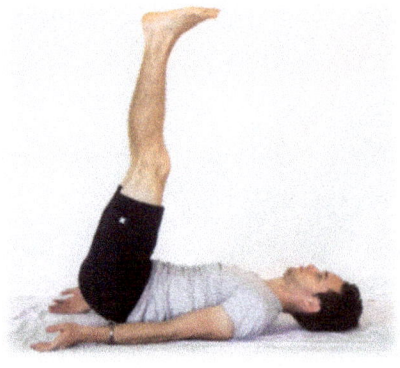

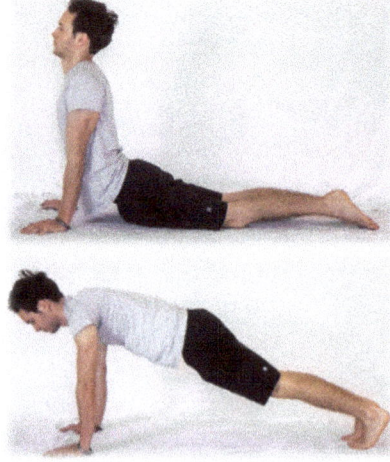

6) Cobra pose with Long Deep Breath for **1 minute.**

7) Dynamic cobra
Inhale move to front platform exhale move into cobra. **26 times.**

8) Cobra pose and hold the asana with Breath of Fire for **1 minute.**

9) Cobra with pranayam. Inhale look over left shoulder at heels, exhale look over right shoulder at heels. **1 - 3 minutes.**

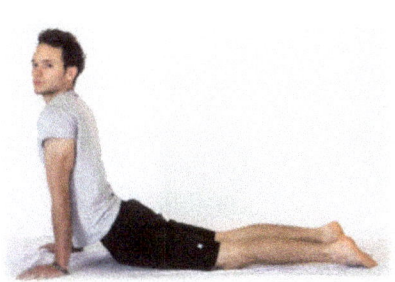

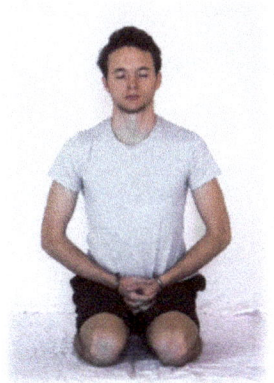

10) Sit on heels. Meditate **3 minutes.**

11) Sit in between heels in celibate pose. Interlace the hands index fingers point up. Pull navel back chant 'Sat' then release and chant 'Nam', continue Sat Kriya for **3 - 8 minutes.**

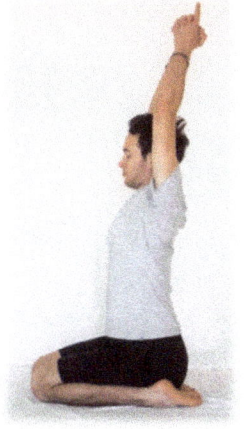

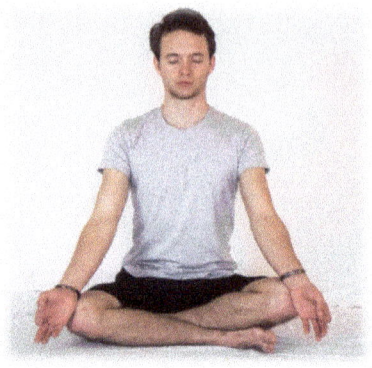

12) Easy pose, hands in gyan mudra on knees. Meditate for **3 to 11 minutes.**

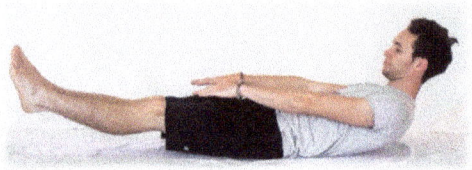

13) Stretch pose, on back raise legs, arms and head 6 inches off the floor and hold with Long Deep Breathing. **1 minute.**

14) Corpse pose **2 - 5 minutes.**

15) Sit in easy pose. Arms above head, fingers interlaced index fingers point up. Inhale, mentally chant 'SAT' and visualize the energy rising up the spine, exhale and me ntally chant 'NAM' and visualize the energy going out the top of the head. **3 – 11 minutes**.

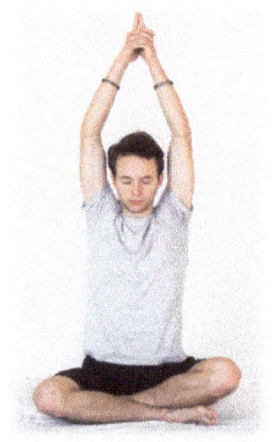

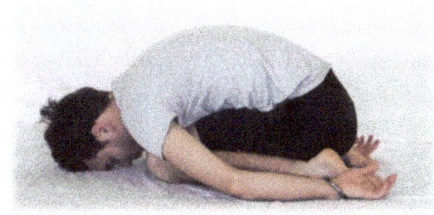

16) GuruPranam, sit on heels, bring forehead to the ground with arms by the sides. Chant 'ONG' long and slow for **1 - 3 minutes.**

17) Sit with left leg extended out in front and right foot on top of the left thigh, hold left big toe with left hand, reach around the back with the right hand and try and hold the right big toe. Look to the right over the shoulder with long deep breathing.
2 - 5 minutes.

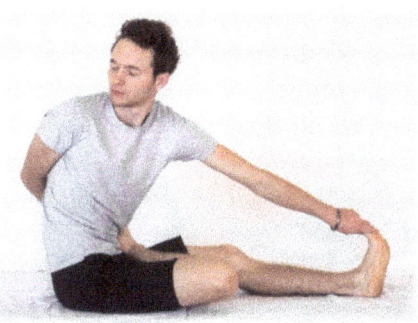

Reverse sides and repeat for **2 - 5 minutes.**

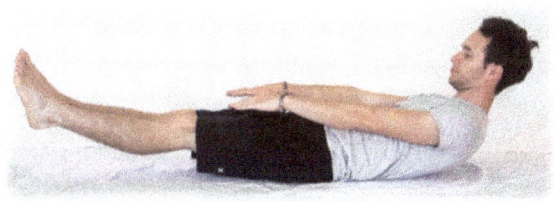

18) Stretch pose. On back, left arms, legs, head 6 inches of ground, hold posture with Long Deep Breathing for **30 seconds**. Relax on back for **1 minute.** Repeat three times.

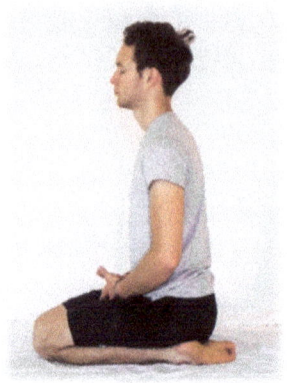

19) Sit on heels. Meditate on the etheric silver cord, the inside of spine from the root to 5th chakra.
2 - 5 minutes.

20) Sit on heels, Sat Kriya for **3 - 8 minutes**.

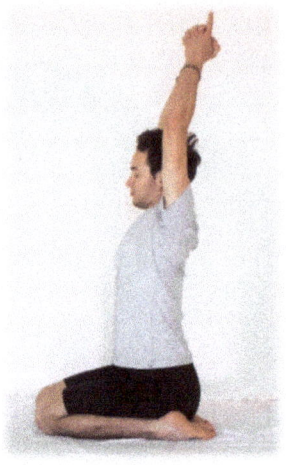

21) Shavasana.

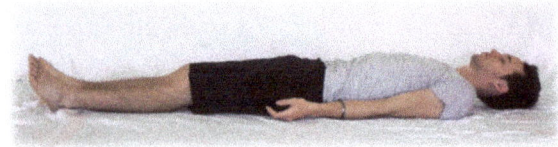

3rd BODY
Kundalini Yoga Meditation
Meditation to Give Balance through Touch

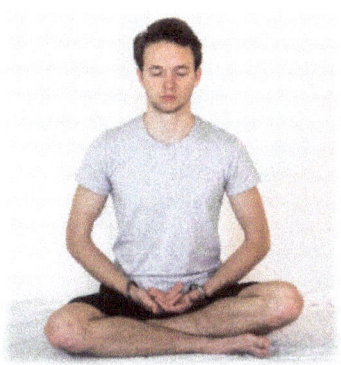

Sit in easy pose, palms face up and interlace the fingers so they point up and don't touch each other. Thumbs point away from body, fingers point up and don't touch each other.

- *To increase masculine energy interlace fingers pointing up with left little finger closest to the body.*
- *To increase feminine energy interlace fingers with right little finger closest to body.*

Place tongue into soft palate at roof of mouth. Eyes focus at tip of nose.

Inhale in 4 parts and mentally chant: 'SA, TA, NA, MA', exhale 1 part and mentally chant 'WAHE GURU'. **11-31 minutes.**

To end; inhale roll eyes up internally towards 3rd eye hold for as long as possible then exhale and relax.

4th BODY
Kundalini Yoga Kriya
Cup of Prayer

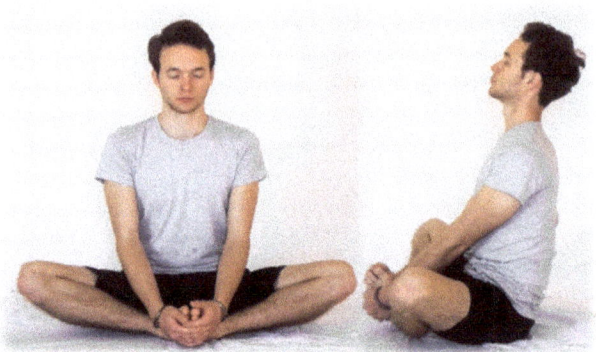

1) Sit in easy pose. Bring feet together in groin, hold feet with hands. Apply a slight neck lock and lean head back with eyes closed and hold with Long Deep Breathing for **3 - 7 minutes.**

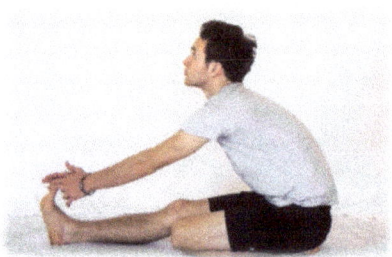

2) Sit on left heel, right leg out straight. Hold right toes with hands and look up to the sky. Long Deep Breathing. **3 - 7 minutes**. <u>Do not reverse.</u>

3) Sit in full lotus, or easy pose. Hands in fists, lift body off ground, lean head back. **3 – 7 minutes.**

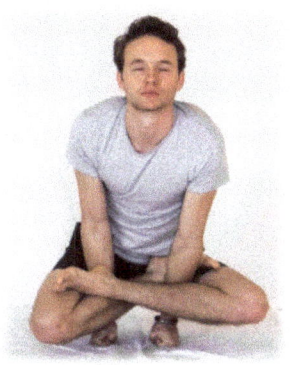

*Modification: sit in easy pose with hands by sides and lift body off ground and lean head back a little bit.

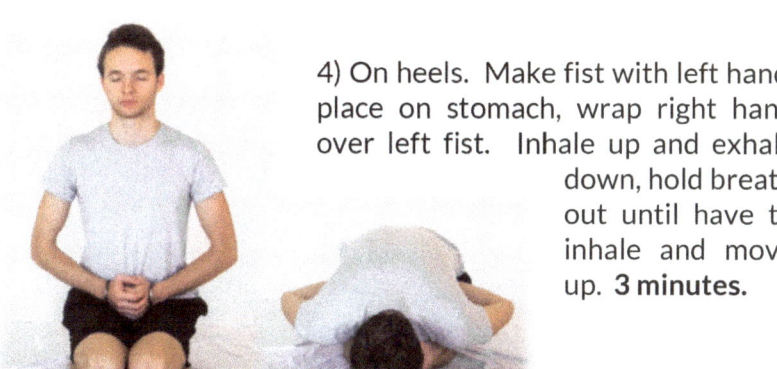

4) On heels. Make fist with left hand, place on stomach, wrap right hand over left fist. Inhale up and exhale down, hold breath out until have to inhale and move up. **3 minutes.**

5) Easy pose. Hands relaxed. Inhale with whistle and make sound 'WHOO', exhale chant 'LAAA' to open heart chakra.
3 minutes.

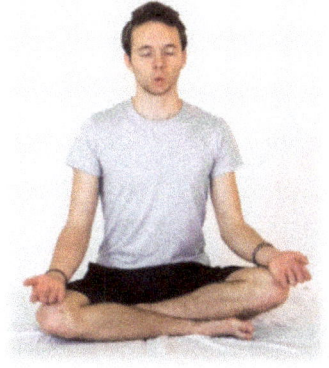

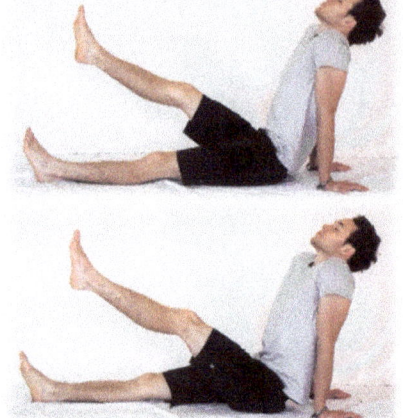

6. Sit with legs out in front. Hands by sides on ground, fingers point back. Raise right leg chant ' RA', raise left leg chant 'MA'. Head in line with spine.

Keep heart open and extended continue for **11 minutes.**

6) Sit in easy pose. Hands in Gyan Mudra on knees. Meditate in silence for as long as you like.

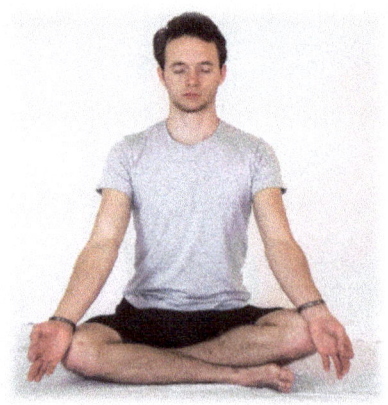

4th BODY
Kundalini Yoga Meditation
Cup of Prayer

Meditation to Gain Healing Power

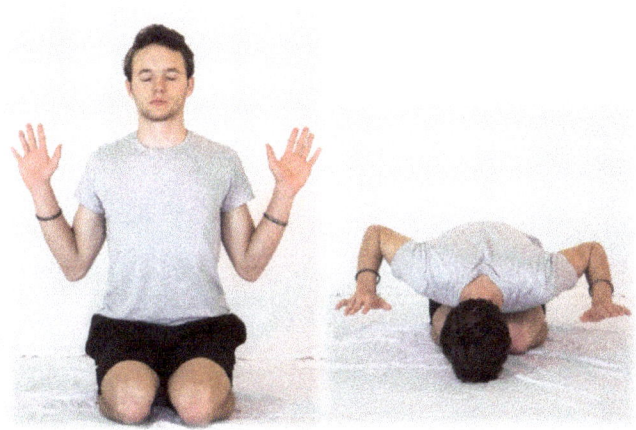

Sit on heels. Elbows in sides, hands raised ear high as if taking an oath. Palms face forward. Focus at brow point. Bow to ground WITHOUT hands touching ground and chant from navel 'WAHE'. Rise up and chant 'GURU'.

With each repetition of the mantra contract mulbandh tighter and tighter.

To end, inhale, hold and meditate on center of palms.
7 – 11 minutes.

5th BODY
Kundalini Yoga Kriya
Half Balance

1) Easy pose. Inhale turn head to left, exhale turn head to right. **2 minutes.**

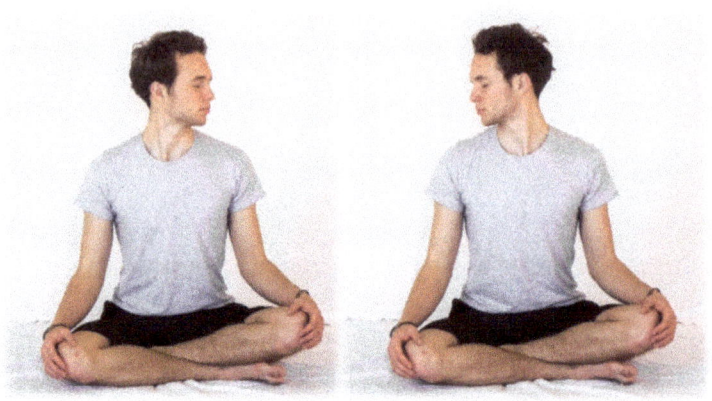

2) Sit on heels. Hands on shoulders, elbows in line with shoulders. Inhale then exhale and apply mulbandh.

Contract muscles at rectum, sex organs and navel in this wave like motion and hold for as long as you can then inhale and continue to apply mulbandh on the exhale for **2 minutes.**

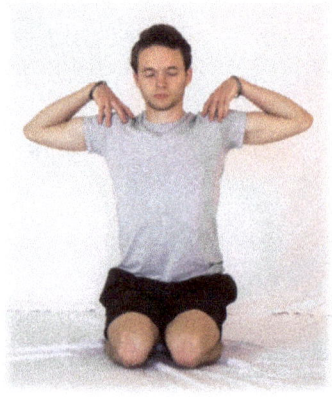

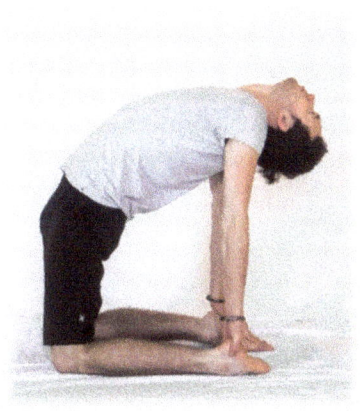

3) Camel pose. Sit on heels, come up on knees, press thighs forward and lean back. Hands hold ankles. Hold asana with Breath of Fire **1 minute.**

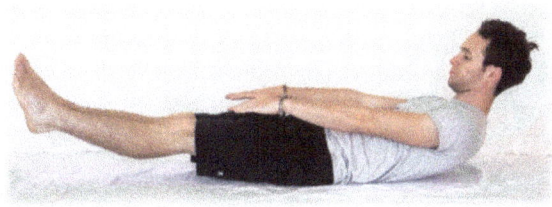

4) Stretch pose. Lie on back, lift arms, legs and head 6 inches of floor. Breath of Fire for **1 minute.**

5) Crow pose. Stand then squat down, arms out and hands interlaced. Stay in crow pose with Breath of Fire for **3 minutes.**

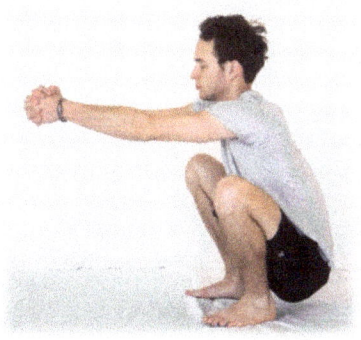

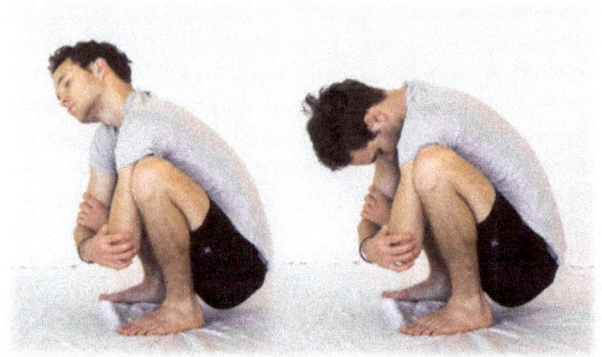

6) Crow pose arms crossed. Roll neck in one direction with regular breathing for **1 minute** then reverse direction and roll the neck for **1 minute**.

7) Cobra pose. Lie on stomach, hands under shoulders, straighten arms. Figure 8 neck rolls, drop head forward and roll to left shoulder then back and then to the right shoulder for **1 minute** then reverse direction for **another minute**.

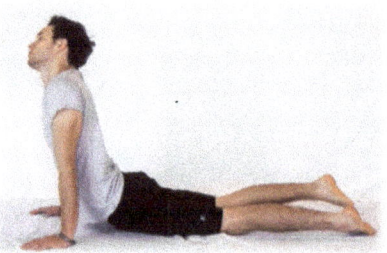

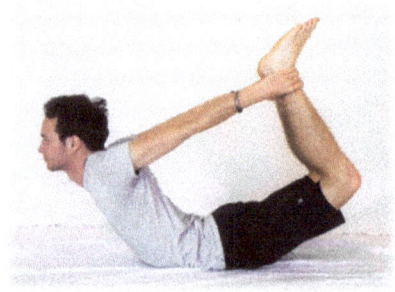

8) Bow pose. On stomach, chin on ground, reach back and hold ankles and lift up. Continue figure 8 neck rolls in one direction for **1 minute** and in other direction for **1 minute**.

9) Lie on back. Arms by sides, raise alternate arms straight up on inhale, exhale down. **1 minute.**

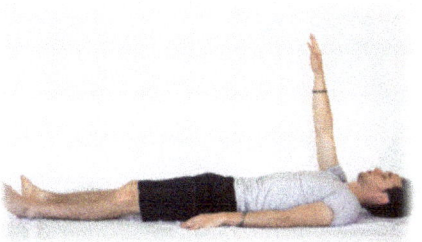

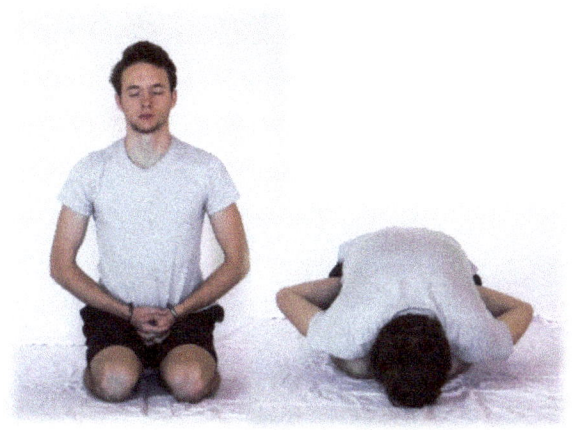

10. Sit on heels. Hands in Venus lock in lap. Inhale up then exhale bow down. Continue dynamic bowing with Long Deep Breathing for **3 minutes.**

11) Cobra pose. On stomach, hands under shoulders, chin on ground, raise up and hold with Long Deep Breathing for **2 minutes.**

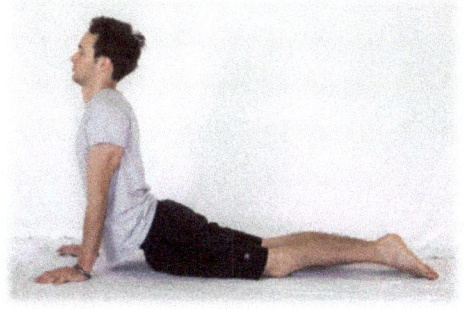

12) Lie on belly, arms out front and stretch whole body for **30 seconds.**

13) Shavasana for **11 minutes.**

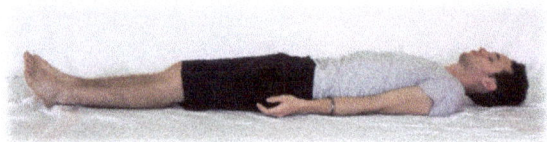

5th BODY
Kundalini Yoga Meditation
Half Balance

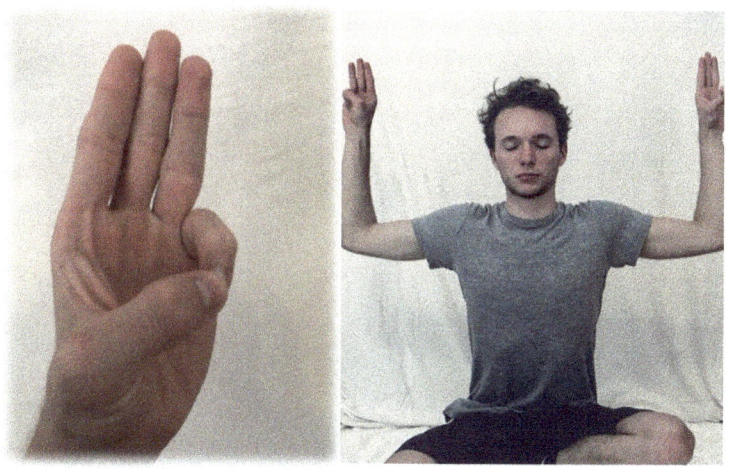

Sit in easy pose. Arms up in Egyptian pose. Thumb of each hand presses little finger into pad of hand. Index, middle and ring fingers extend straight up. Palms face forward. Focus at brow point.

Mentally chant:

> *"SAT NAM SAT NAM SAT NAM*
> *SAT NAM SAT NAM SAT NAM WAHE GURU"*

11 minutes.

6ᵗʰ BODY
Kundalini Yoga Kriya
Person at Prayer

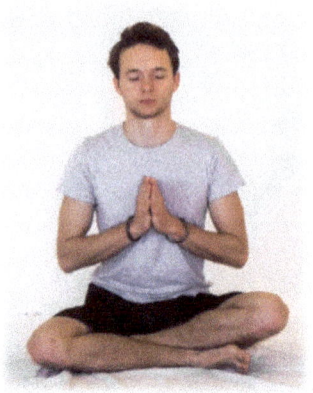

1) Sit in easy pose with hands in prayer pose at the heart. **Breath of Fire. 3 minutes.**

2) Easy pose. Lightly touch back of neck with all 10 fingers, lean back slightly, hold and balance at 3ʳᵈ eye. Long Deep Breathing **1 – 3 minutes.**

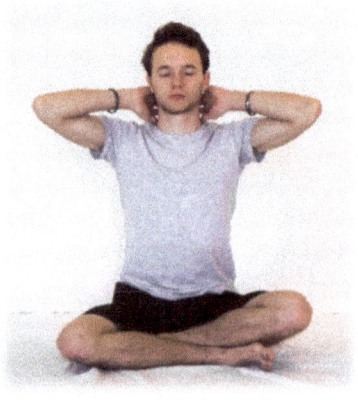

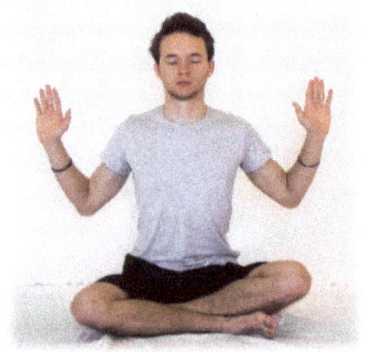

3) Easy pose. Hands in prayer pose and chant 'WAHE GURU' then move hands out to the sides (as if taking a vow) and chant 'WAHE GURU'. Move from finite to infinite. Continue for **1 – 3 minutes.**

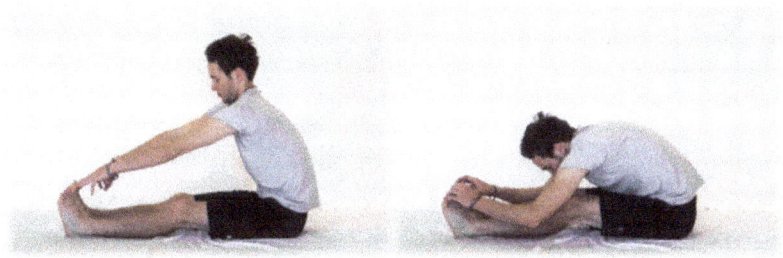

4) Sit with legs out in front. Hold feet and pull spine straight. Inhale up, exhale down and apply neck and diaphragm locks. Continue dynamic front leg stretch with bandhas applied only on exhale for **3 minutes**.

5) On all fours. Extend right leg up 60 degrees with forehead on ground, and ONLY the palms on the ground next to the head, keep elbows close to sides.

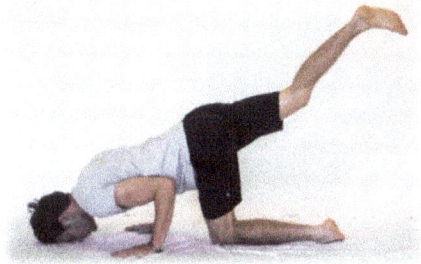

Breathe from sole of extended foot into the 3rd eye. Long deep Breath for **2 ½ minutes** then **30 seconds** of Breath of Fire. Repeat on other side.

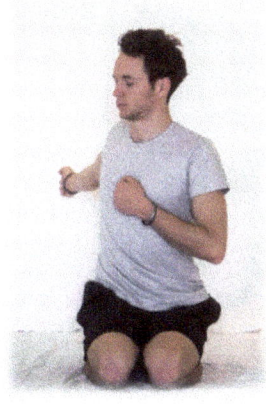

6) Sit on heels. Hands in soft fists at heart. Inhale and turn upper body left as left arm extends back and right hand stays at heart, exhale as right arm extends back and left hand is at heart. Continue dynamic side-to-side movement with arms. **3 minutes.**

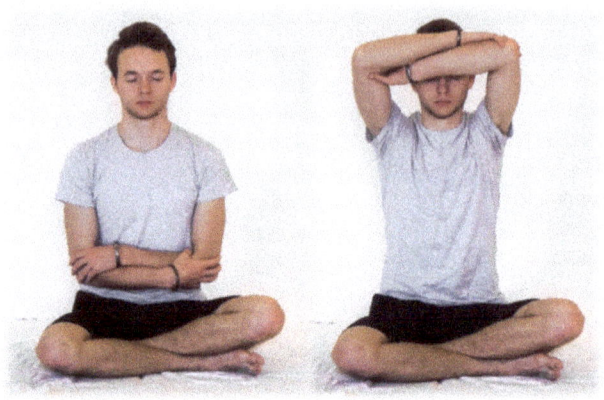

7) Easy pose. Fold arms in front of heart, right hand holds left elbow, left hand hold right elbow. Move arms down to navel, chant 'SAT' move arms to 3rd eye chant 'NAM'. Observe the fluctuations at the silver cord. **7 ½ - 11 minutes.**

8) Shavasana.

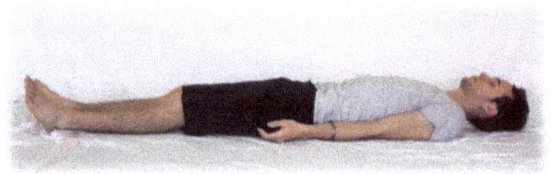

6ᵗʰ BODY
Kundalini Yoga Meditation
Person at Prayer

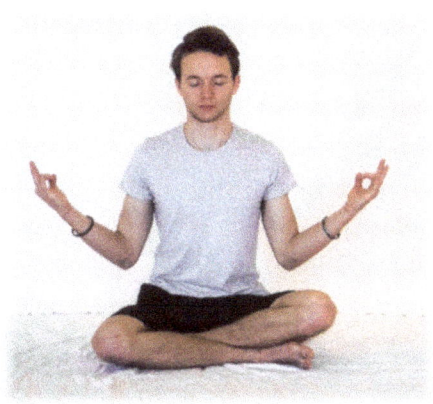

Easy pose. Elbows by sides, not touching the body. Forearms up 60 degrees. Hands in gyan mudra. Palms face body. Look at brow point.

Chant

*' SAT NAM SAT NAM SAT NAM SAT NAM
SAT NAM SAT NAM WAHE GURU'*

Let the breath find itself. Continue **7 to 31 minutes.**

7th BODY
Kundalini Yoga Kriya
Platform of Elevation

1) Easy pose. Hold right foot, put around back of neck and on left shoulder.

Alternately, hold right foot and lift towards left shoulder as much as possible. Hold for **2 minutes.**

(does not repeat on other side)

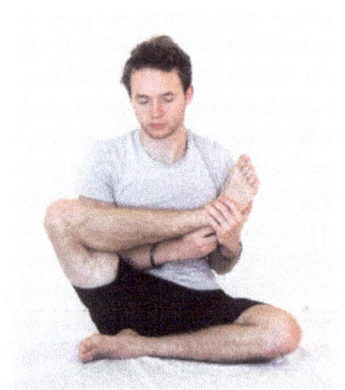

2. Sit on heels. Hands on ground in front of knees. Inhale up and exhale forehead down. Continue bowing for **2 minutes.**

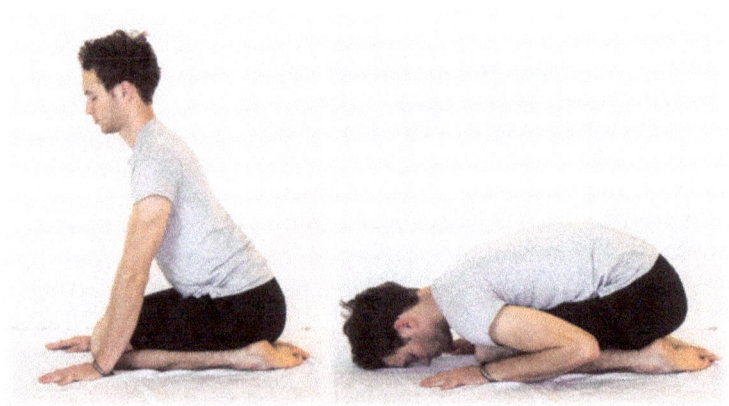

189

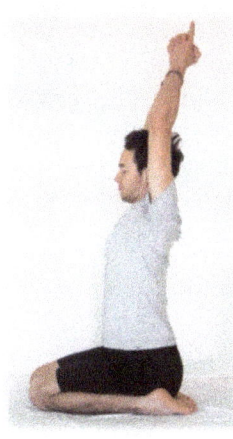

3) Sit on heels. Raise arms and clasp hands together, raise index finger straight up. Chant long 'SAT NAM'. **2 minutes.**

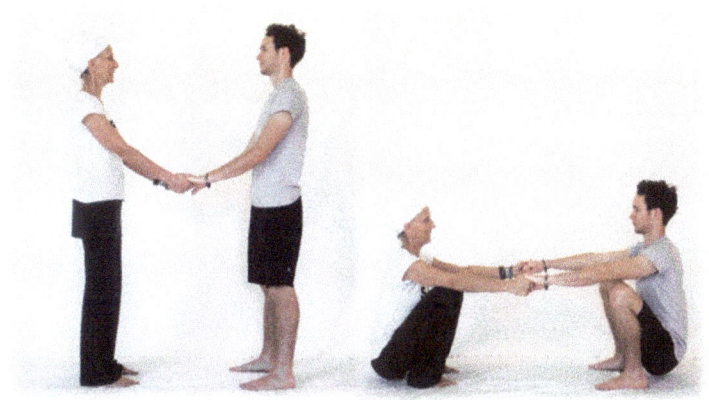

4.) Hold hands with partner (if available). Crow squats: inhale up, exhale down. **2 minutes.**

5) Bridge pose. Sit with hands behind hips. Place feet on ground in front of hips. Lift torso parallel to ground, Let head relax back. Breath of Fire. **2 minutes.**

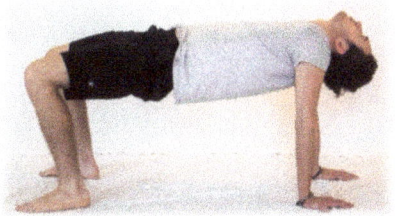

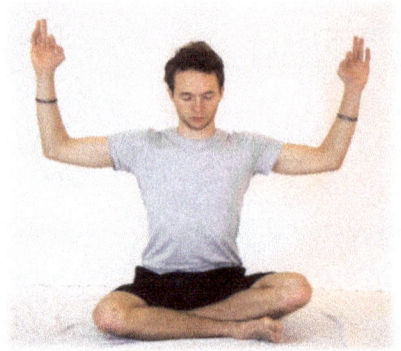

6) Egyptian pose. Easy pose, raise arms, forearms perpendicular to ground, Hands in Gyan Mudra. Breath of Fire. **2 minutes.** Inhale and exhale apply mulbandh.

7) Easy pose. Hands hold shoulders, long deep breathing. **2 minutes.**

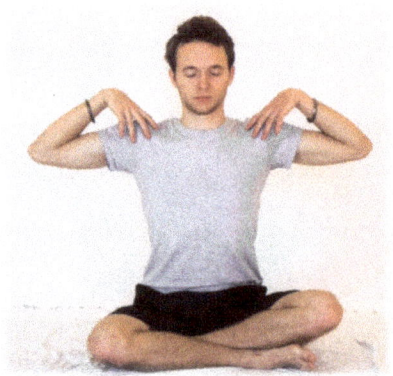

8) Extend both legs out front. Hold feet and relax down. Long deep breathing. **2 minutes.**

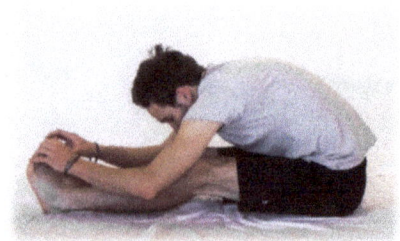

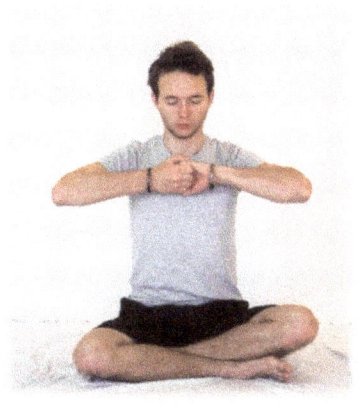

9) Easy pose. Clasp fingers in Bear grip at heart, left faces out, right faces in. Inhale then exhale and apply Mulbandh. **Do this 3 times only**.

10) Easy pose. Close off left nostril and breathe through right nostril only. Continue Long Deep Breathing for **2 minutes** then inhale, exhale apply Mullbandh and relax.

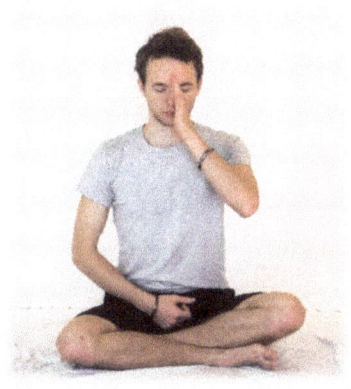

11) Shavasana.

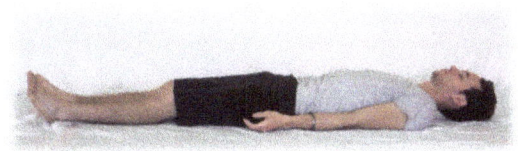

7th BODY
Kundalini Yoga Meditation
Platform of Elevation

Balances sun and moon energies

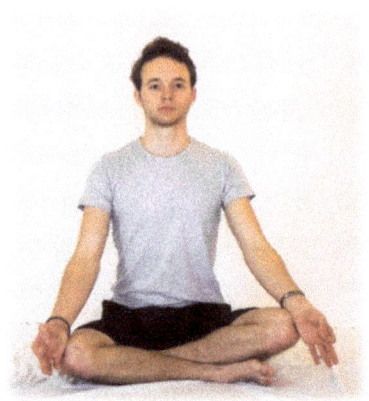

PART 1
Easy pose. Hands in Gyan Mudra on knees. Eyes open gaze straight ahead.

Inhale for 5 seconds, hold 10 seconds, exhale 5 seconds. **11 minutes** to reach a state of Pratyahar.

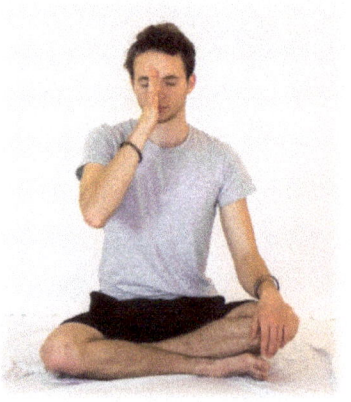

PART 2
Sit in easy pose. Inhale through left nostril and hold for 45 seconds. Exhale through right nostril in 4 strokes for **7 minutes.**

PART 3
Inhale through left nostril and hold for 45 seconds. Exhale through right nostril in 8 strokes. **8 minutes.**

8th BODY
Kundalini Yoga Kriya
Finite to Infinite

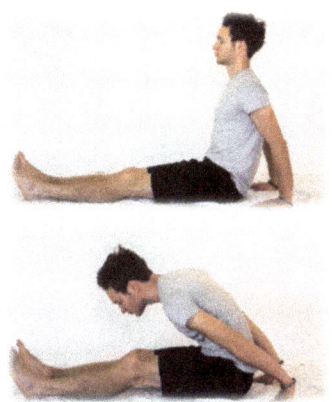

1) Sit with legs extended out front, hands by hips on floor. Inhale sit up straight, exhale lead with the heart and lean forward to floor. Continue movement for **2 minutes.**

2) On back. Arms by sides, or the modification is with hands under hips. Each position with long deep breathing for **1 minute**.

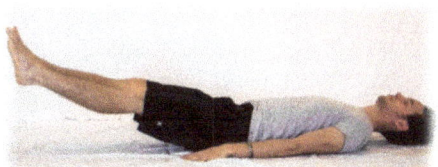

Raise legs to 6 inches and hold,

Raise legs 1 inch and hold,

Raise legs 2 inches and hold,

Raise legs 3 inches and hold,

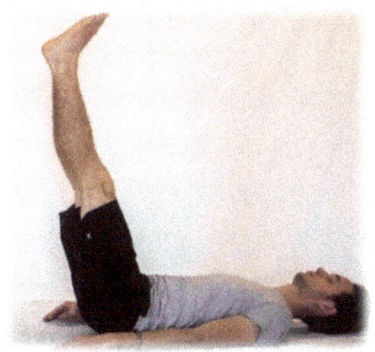

Raise legs to 90 degrees and hold.

3) Plow pose. Lie on back and raise legs up and to the ground over the head. Support lower back with hands. Long Deep Breathing. **3 minutes.**

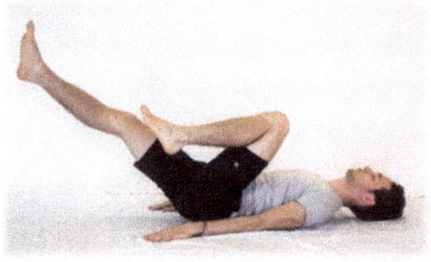

4) On back 2 leg bicycle. Lift legs 18 inches and alternately pull in to chest and extend out. Continue for **5 minutes.**

5) Relax on back. **3 minutes.**

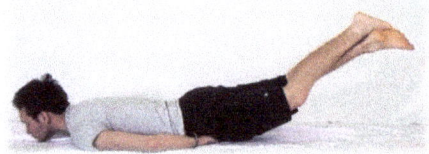

6) Locust pose. On stomach. Chin on ground. Hands in fists inside groin, cross the legs and lift only legs of ground. Hold with regular breath, **3 minutes.**

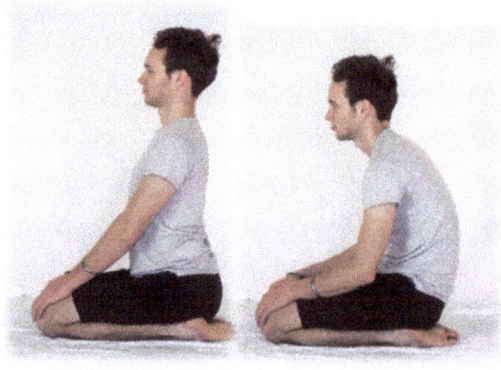

7) Rock pose. Sit on heels. Hands on thighs. Hold head still, inhale flex spine forward, exhale flex spine back. Continue spine flex for **2 minutes.**

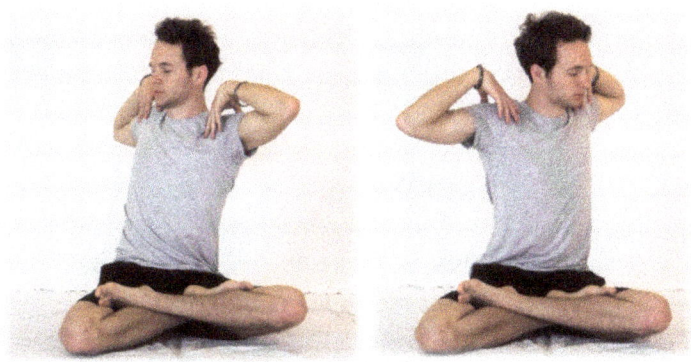

8) Sit in full lotus, modification: sit in easy pose, place hands on shoulders, inhale twist left, exhale twist right. **2 minutes.**

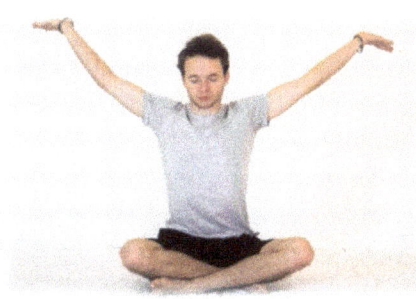

9) Easy pose. Raise arms 60 degrees with palms flat as if holding a tray and fingers point to sides. Breath of Fire **2 minutes.**

To end, inhale bring palms together, exhale relax arms down.

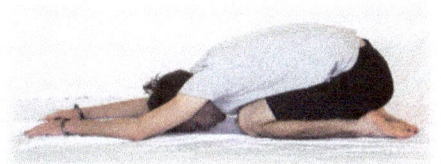

10) Gurpranam. Sit on heels, bring forehead to ground, arms extended in front, palms down. Relax. **2 minutes.**

11) Easy pose. Hands on knees. Inhale and raise both shoulders up, exhale down. Continue with rapid movement for **3 minutes.**

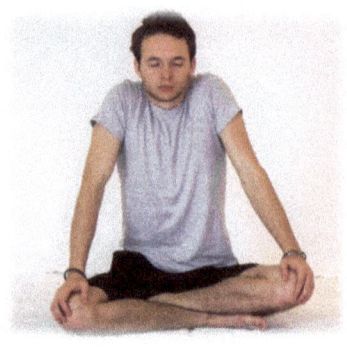

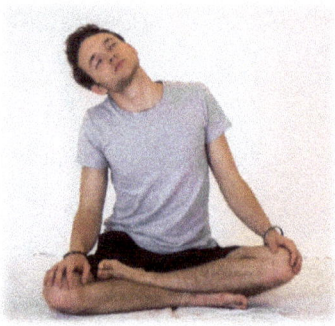 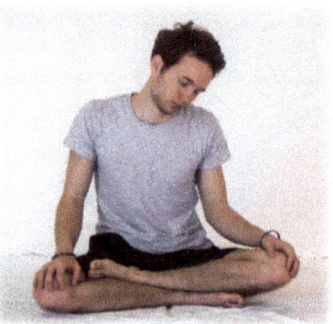

12) Easy pose. Figure 8 neck rolls from shoulder to shoulder. **1 minute** one direction, **1 minute** other direction.

13) Easy pose.
Meditate in silence **3 minutes.**

14) Sat Kriya **5 minutes.**

15) Shavasana.

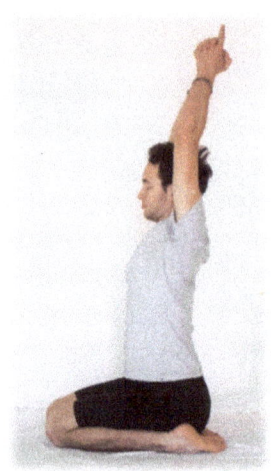

8ᵗʰ BODY
Kundalini Yoga Meditation
Finite to Infinite

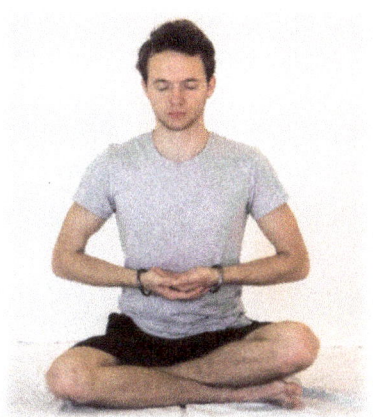

SARAVASUD *that which corrects everything*

Sit in easy pose with hands in Buddha mudra. Right hand in left, thumb tips touch. Hold mudra against solar plexus.
Focus at 3ʳᵈ eye.

Chant:

> *'HARI HARI HARI HARI HARI HARI HAR'*
> lift the diaphragm on the last HAR.

Project green light from brow, radiate healing energy.
11 minutes.

Do this meditation for:
- Dealing with others with mental imbalances.
- Self healing.
- Stability in relationships.
- Bringing in "green' energy, prosperity.

9th BODY
Kundalini Yoga Kriya
God and Blessings

1) a) Lie on back. Lift both legs 6 inches with long deep breathing for **1 minute.**

Modification: place hands palms down under buttocks for support when lifting the legs. Relax **1 minute.**

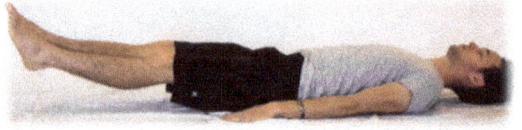

b) Lift both legs 2 inches with long deep breathing for 1 minute. Relax **1 minute.**

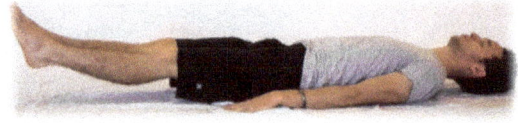

c) Lift both legs 3 inches with long deep breathing for 1 minute. Relax **1 minute.**

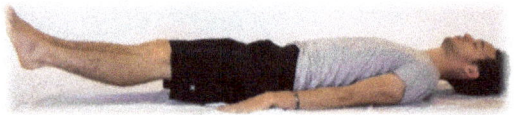

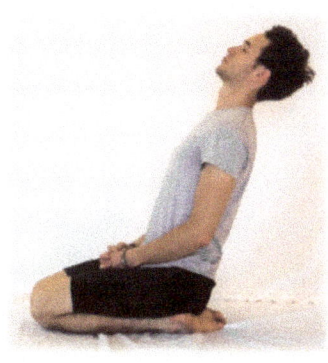

2) Sit on heels. Place hands in Venus lock in lap. Inhale lean back 60 degrees, exhale bow down to ground. Continue SLOW bowing movement for **10 minutes.**

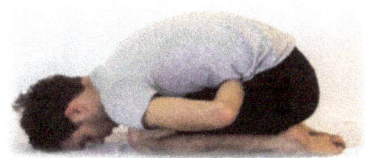

3) One side life nerve stretch. Sit with legs extended, bring one foot on opposite thigh. Relax in downward stretch with long deep breathing. **5 minutes.** Switch sides and repeat for **5 minutes.**

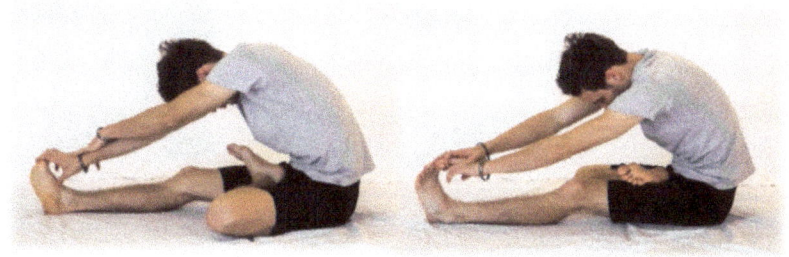

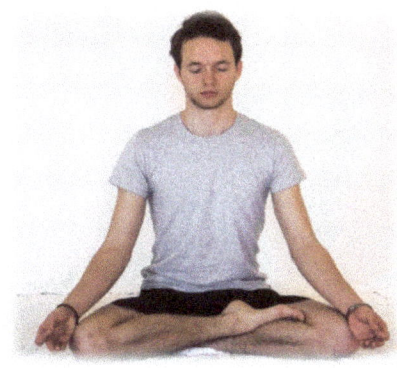

4) Sidhasan. Sit on left heel with heel in perineum. Tuck toes from right foot in behind left knee. Hands on knees in Gyan Mudra. Chant long 'SAT NAM'. Continue for **3 - 5 minutes.**

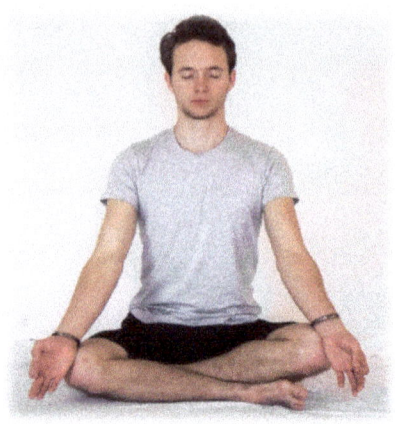

5) Easy pose. Hands on knees in Gyan Mudra. Meditate on tip of nose with Long Deep Breathing. **3 minutes.**

To end, inhale and exhale apply mulbandh. Repeat 3 times.

6) Shavasana.

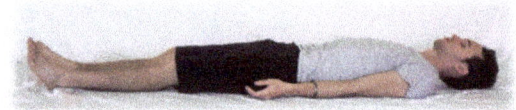

9th BODY
Kundalini Yoga Meditation
God and Blessings

There are 5 parts to this meditation!

PART 1

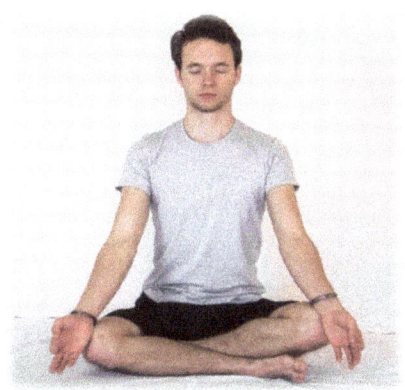

Sit in easy pose. Hands in Gyan Mudra on knees. Focus at tip of nose. Long Deep Breathing from navel. Inhale mentally chant: 'WAHE' exhale: 'GURU'. **31 minutes.**

PART 2
Shavasana: **31 minutes.**

PART 3
Sit in easy pose with each foot tucked in between the calves and thighs.

Inhale hold the breath then apply Mulbandh and pump stomach for as long as you can, exhale, then inhale and continue   pumping the stomach on the inhale only for **5 minutes.**

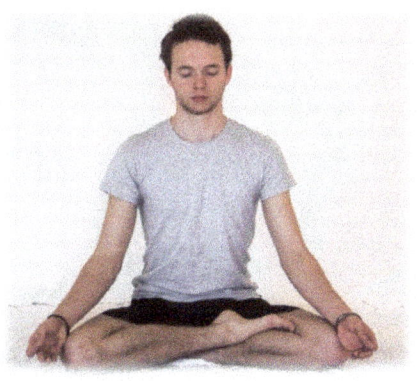

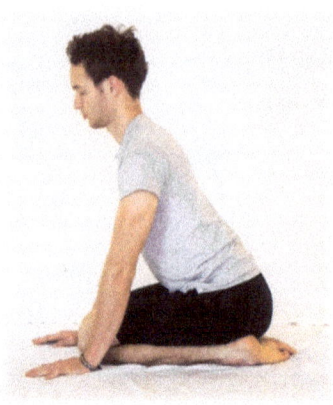

PART 4
On heels or in easy pose, put both hands on floor, inhale flex spine forward, exhale flex spine back. Continue for **5 minutes.**

PART 5
Sit in silence and meditate for **5 minutes.**

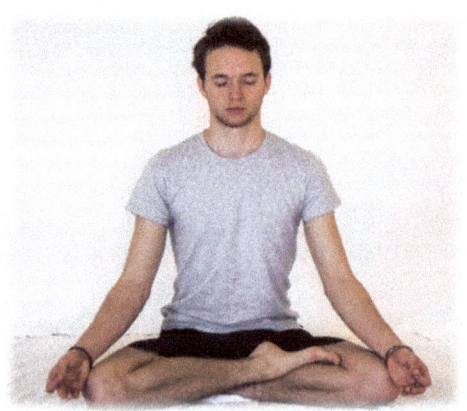

10th BODY
Kundalini Yoga Kriya
Reach for Infinity

1) Easy pose. Raise arms 60 degrees, palms flat facing up. Breath of Fire.
3 minutes.

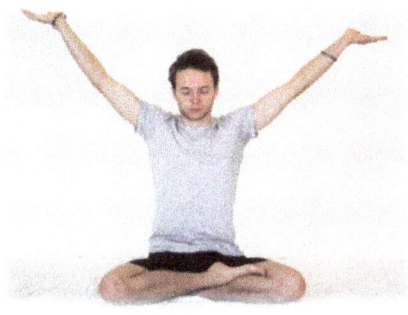

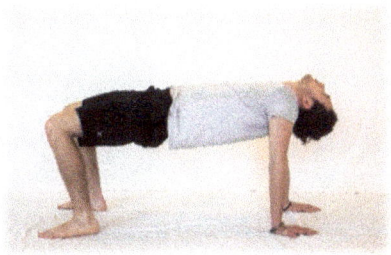

2) Bridge pose. Sit, lean back on arms, place feet by buttocks and raise body up parallel to ground. Relax head back. Breath of Fire.
3 minutes.

3) Easy pose. Raise arms 60 degrees with hands in Gyan Mudra. Breath of Fire.
2 minutes.

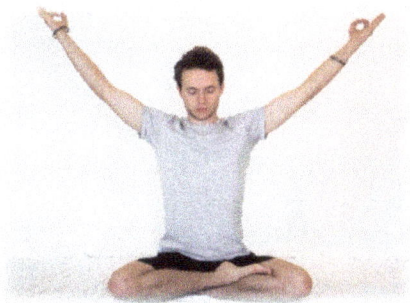

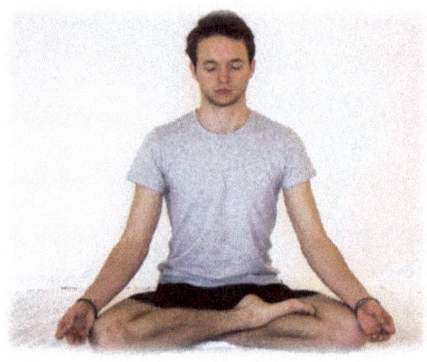

4) Easy pose. Meditate on brow. **11 minutes.**

5) Easy pose. Raise arms 60 degrees with hands in Gyan Mudra. Breath of Fire. **2 minutes**.

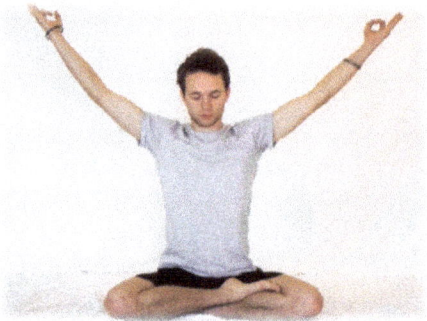

6) Easy pose. Hold shoulders with Long Deep Breathing. **3 minutes.**

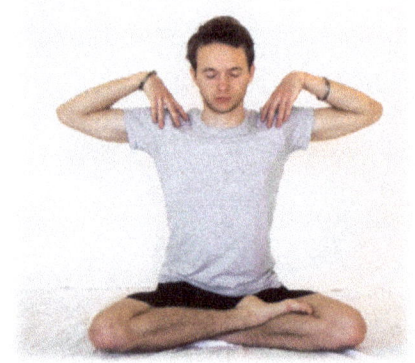

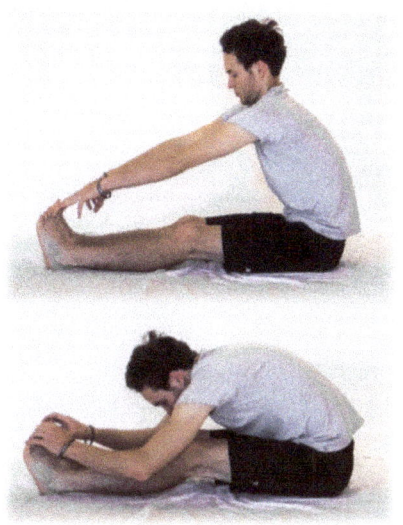

7) Dynamic 2 leg life nerve stretch. Extend legs out in front reach forward hold toes. Inhale up, exhale down. **2 minutes.**

8) Sit with legs out in front. Lean back on hands. Alternate leg lifts. Inhale raise one leg to 60 degrees, exhale down, inhale raise other leg to 60 degrees, exhale down. Keep heart extended forward and continue for **1 minute.**

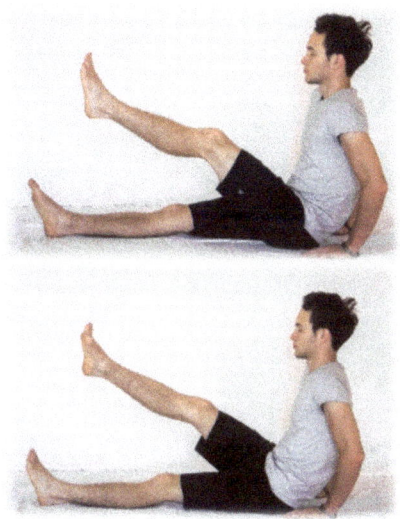

9) Shavasana.

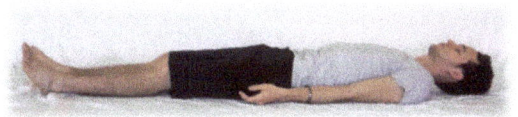

206

10th BODY
Kundalini Yoga Meditation
Reach for Infinity

Do this meditation subtly and delicately in a quiet environment.

Sit in easy pose. Both hands palms down between heart and throat.

Place the INSIDE edge of 1st section of left pinky (Mercury) against the INSIDE edge of the 1st section of the index (Jupiter) finger. Keep firm pressure, these fingers will move 45 degrees away from the other fingers.

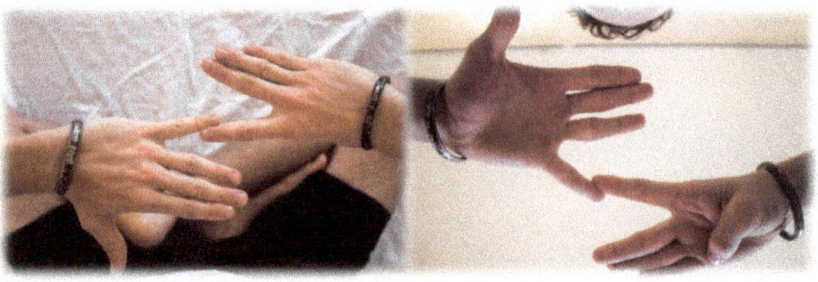

Other fingers of hands are straight, parallel to ground and together.

Right thumb pulls into the right palm and points away from body. Left thumb points towards the body and is away from hand.

No bend at the wrists. Forearm parallel to ground.

Eyes closed.

Inhale and chant:
> 'GOBINDE GOBINDE GOBINDE
> GOBINDE GOBINDE GOBINDE GOBINDAH'
> *4 times per breath.*

11 – 31 minutes.

11th BODY
Kundalini Yoga Kriya
Unto Infinity

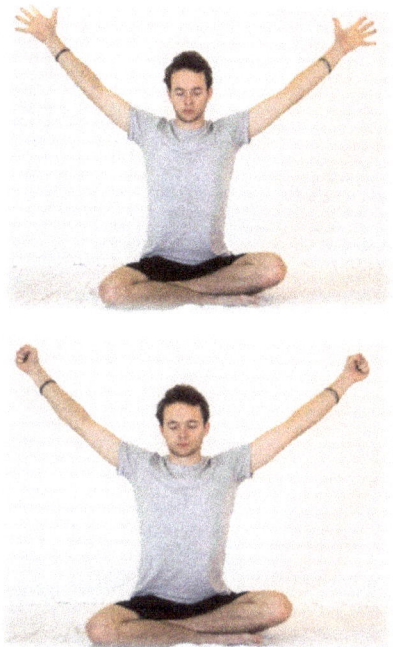

1) Easy pose. Raise arms 60 degrees. Make fists on the inhale and open hands on the exhale with Long Deep Breathing for **1 minute** and then with Breath of Fire for **2 minutes**, and continue to open and close the fists on the inhale and exhale!

2) Sit on heels. Spine flex, inhale forward, and lift both shoulders, exhale flex back and release shoulders. Feel the brilliance of the sushmana nadi. Continue dynamic spine flex for **2 minutes.**

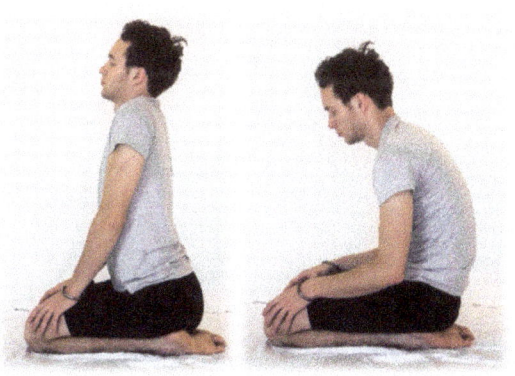

3) Meditate in easy pose for **1 – 3 min**.

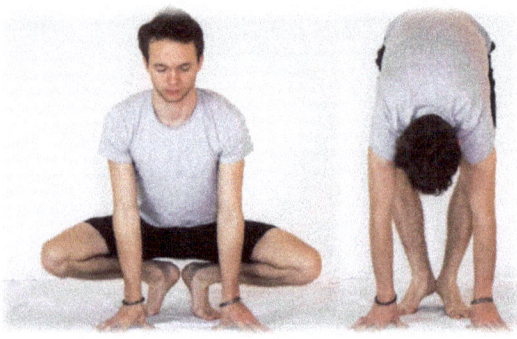

4) Frog pose **26x**. Squat with heels off ground, hands on ground in front, inhale straighten legs with head down, exhale squat down, keep heels off ground.

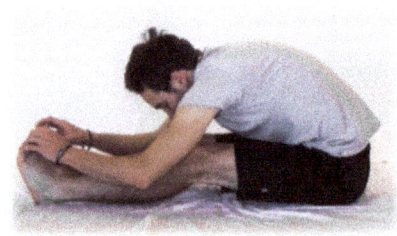

5) Life nerve stretch. Sit with legs stretched out in front, hold toes and pull back gently, then leading with the heart relax down and hold with Long Deep Breathing for **1 minute.**

6) Sit with legs stretched out in front. Hands by hips on ground, lift both legs 60 degrees with any breath. **2-3 minutes.**

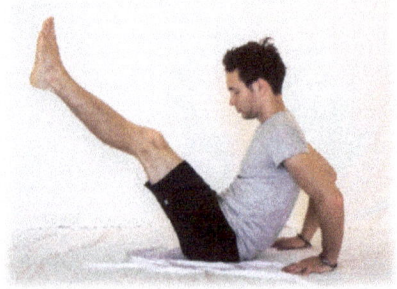

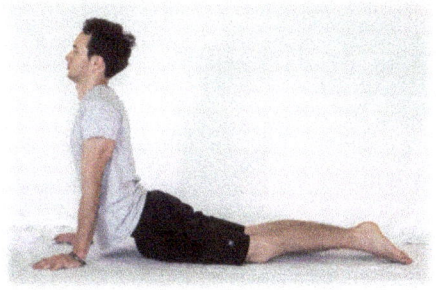

7) Cobra pose, lie on stomach place hands under shoulders on ground with fingers spread wide, straighten the arms and raise up, hold with light Breath of Fire **3 – 5 minutes.**

8) Shoulder stand. Lie on back and raise legs, hands support low back. Long Deep Breath for **3 minutes.**

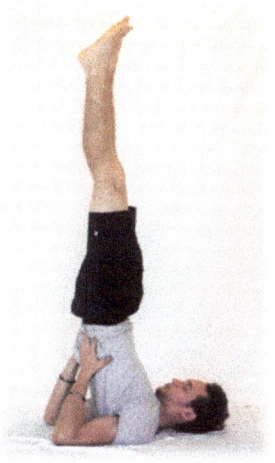

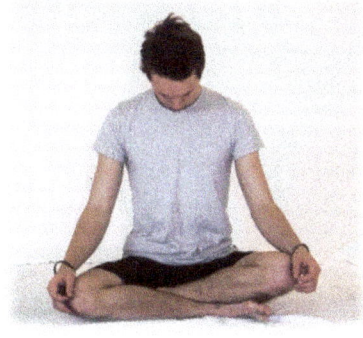

9) Easy pose. Drop head forward and roll head all around in one direction for **1 minute** and reverse for **1 minute.**

10) Easy pose. Inhale and turn head to the left, exhale turn to the right continue for **3 minutes.**

11) Shavasana

210

11ᵗʰ BODY
Kundalini Yoga Meditation
Unto Infinity

This meditation produces the radiance needed to carry the soul through the void at the time of death. If your thumbs heat up, keep the hands in fists and place them on knees until they cool down and then slowly open the fists.

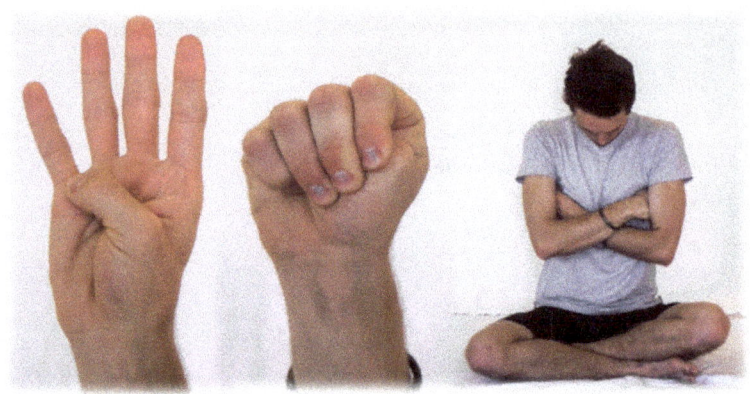

Sit in easy pose. Place each thumb on the mercury mound (base of little finger) and then make a fist with each hand. Place fists with thumbs folded inside, in opposite arm pits. Right arm over left arm. Pressure will be felt on fists.

Bend head down with chin on the chest.

Eyes open 1/10ᵗʰ.
Inhale: Mentally vibrate 'WA' for 2 seconds
Hold: Mentally vibrate 'HE' for 2 seconds
Exhale: Mentally vibrate 'GURU' for 4 seconds

3 - 11 minutes.

GLOSSARY

BANDHAS: Three Internal Locks to help bring order to the complex patterns of internal energies and to enlist the body as a tool for the development of self-awareness. These locks—the throat lock, stomach lock, and root lock—are fundamental practices of yoga that can be learned relatively easily and then further refined with practice.

DRISTHI: the method of gazing at a focal point in yoga practice.

JIWAN MUKTA: someone who has gained the self-awareness to remain unaffected by the polarities of life and who lives with an inner sense of freedom.

PATANJALI RISHI - The compiler of the Yoga Sutras, a text on yoga theory and practice, and a notable scholar of the Samkhya school of Hindu philosophy. He is estimated to have lived between 2nd century BCE to 4th century BCE. The Sutras are one of the most important texts in the Hindu tradition and are the foundation of all Yoga.

PRAKIRTI: the prime material energy of which all matter is composed.

PRANA & APANA – Through their exploration of the body and breath, the ancient yogis discovered that prana (life force energy) could be further subdivided into energetic components they called Vayus (winds). The five Vayus of prana all have very subtle yet distinct energetic qualities, including specific functions and directions of flow. The yogis were able to control and cultivate these Vayus by simply bringing their focus and awareness to them. Through this conscious control and cultivation they were not only able to create optimal health and well-being, but were able to activate the primordial Kundalini energy to obtain states of enlightened Samadhi.

The two most important Vayus are Prana and Apana. Prana is situated between the base of the heart and the neck and its energy pervades the chest region. The flow of Prana is inwards and upward.

Apana–Vayu is situated below the navel and its energy pervades the lower abdomen. The flow of Apana is downwards and out.

PUJA – a devotional action.

SAMSKARAS: the subtle impressions of past actions.

TAPASYA - is a Sanskrit word that literally means "generation of heat and energy." It is a practical spiritual discipline that involves deep meditation, austerity/moderation, self-discipline, and efforts to reach Self-realization. Yogis practice tapasya for Self Realization.

There are three types of tapasya: tapasya of the body, tapasya of the speech, and tapasya of the mind. Disciplined and concentrated practice of yoga is a form of tapasya. Tapasya can also be practiced through meditation and/or fasting.

Further explanations can be found on our website at www.purestpotential.com

APPENDIX

AFFIRMATIONS

For many years I wondered why people who were disciplined in their practice of yoga seemed so stuck. Many would come to us complaining that they just weren't achieving the progress they had imagined. As we talked it became clear that they had the goal of becoming a yogi, but had failed to define what that meant. No wonder they felt frustrated, because there was no clarity about what the realization of the practice would feel like, taste like, be like. This started our research into yogic and spiritual literature for clear goals and affirmations created by yogis to confirm the purpose for their spiritual practice. Well, they had tremendous clarity, and we found many! This clarity of the experience of self-realization was the "it" that most people had not defined. The honesty, and the devotion were there, but the clarity of what that experience would give was lacking.

The affirmations all described inner qualities such as bliss, joy, and ease. What the ancients had realized is that when these inner qualities become part of your reality they create a base to allow worldly goals to manifest in perfect harmony with your True Self, your Sat Nam. We recommend that you first establish a strong personal daily practice for at least 120 days to change your self-concepts from who you are to who you want to become.

Process:
- o Making the recording using a computer etc:
- o Speak one affirmation at a time.
- o Pause 8 seconds as research has shown a higher impact on retention if this pause is added.
- o Play very simple music in the back ground such as Pachabel Canon in D or your favorite spiritual music.
- o Play this for 24 hours a day.

Some guidelines for creating your own affirmations:
- Add the word now at the end of each affirmation to qualify that "now" is the eternal now.
- State the affirmation in the positive, i.e. do not say: I am getting rid of anger, instead say: I am at peace, now.
- Feel free to redo your affirmations any time you want to!

ALTAR

We have found that personal home altars can be a point of focus for your spirituality, a place where you confirm the mind in compassion and love. It can also be used for healing, manifesting or meditation. The altar symbolizes an area where you honor wisdom, and transformation. Many people have altars out of wood, because the wood's presence gives testimony to the greater cycle of life.

- Items to add to your altar:
    - Pictures of self realized people.
    - Your own picture confirming yourself to be in the company of the realized ones.
    - A mala with 108 beads symbolizing mastery and completion.
    - Objects that make you feel protected and strong.
    - Objects, which represent your divine state, harmony, and serenity.
    - Crystals to represent clarity.
    - Candles to represent enlightenment.
    - Fresh flowers to represent prana.
    - Incense to represent up-liftment.
    - Play specific mantras to confirm the intention for the altar.

When you create your altar let it be dedicated to your own higher self. What you will notice is that as you take time to regularly connect with the altar, you start to unlearn any condescending behavior or language that does not confirm your real identity.

Your words and your actions will become aligned with your higher Self.

We also noticed that the focus for our morning practice changed from trying to get rid of problems to dwelling in bliss. We experienced bliss to be the ultimate state of deep, higher self-love.

BHOJ KRIYA - PRACTICE
Place some almonds in a bowl.

Close your eyes, hands in prayer pose and feel you are going to be blessed. Calm down and empty yourself, so you can receive acceleration, healing, and purity.

Open your eyes and place your hands on your shoulders, right hand on right shoulder, left hand on left shoulder as a sign of strength. Then place your hands on your knees as a sign of strength. Then place your hands over your heart, one hand over the other as a sign of compassion. Then touch your forehead with the palms over the eyes.

Place your hands, palms down, over the food to bless it. Concentrate and bless your own food. Calmly and quietly make a relationship with your food and your spirit. Feel the food piece by piece, touch it, and request of it there is a yoga, a union.

Using all 5 fingers now put an almond in your mouth. Chew it totally until you have twenty-five percent of its size mixed with saliva. Chew it, and don't swallow it. When the food is soft, like jelly, very slowly, swallow it. Then clean the inside of your mouth with your tongue, including around your teeth until there is no food left in your mouth.

Now calmly and quietly in this way eat all the almonds. Keep eating and relating to your food.

The hand you used to eat with, take that hand and bring all the fingers together in a point, and put that in the palm of the other hand. Close that hand like a fist over the food hand. And feel it. Meditate. Continue for 3 minutes.

216

Go wash your hands, face, elbows, eyes, earlobes, above the eyebrows, and the back of the neck. And take the water and sprinkle it on your face.

Eating in this way is a conscious commitment for your health, your vitality, your energy and your prosperity.

COLD SHOWER
Always precede cold showers with an oil massage.

Step by Step 'Abyanga' Oil Massage
This practice balances the air element.

Begin by running some hot water over the bottle to gently warm the oil, or use an oil warmer.

Pour a tablespoon of warm oil onto your scalp and vigorously work in the oil.

Using your fingertips, vigorously massage your head and scalp with small circular strokes, as if you are shampooing. (or you can skip if you don't want to wash your hair).

Move to your face and ears, massaging more gently. Using an open hand to create friction, massage both the front and back of the neck.

Vigorously massage your arms, using a circular motion at the shoulders and elbows, and back-and-forth motions on the upper arms and forearms.

When massaging your chest and stomach, use a gentle circular motion and a straight up-and-down motion over the breastbone.

After applying a bit of oil to both hands, gently reach around to the back and spine and massage them as well as you can without straining.

Vigorously massage your legs as you did your arms, using circular motions at the ankles and knees, back-and-forth motions on the long parts.

After massaging your legs, spend extra time on your feet.

Using the open part of your hand, massage vigorously back and forth over the soles of the feet.

Keeping a thin, almost imperceptible film of oil on the body is considered very beneficial for toning the skin and warming the muscles throughout the day.

Cold Shower
It is recommended that a woman wear undershorts that cover her thighs while she is in the shower. This protects the sex nerve and the femur (thigh bone) from the sudden changes in temperature. (The femur regulates the production of calcium in the body and is very sensitive to temperature.)

After the massage, step into the shower. Let the cold water strike your body while you briskly massage the water into the skin, step out of the water and continue to massage the skin.

Then step back in, and be sure to stand under the spray and allow the breasts to be massaged by the water; continue massaging your entire body, step out again and repeat this process three or five minutes until you feel warm—even though the water is still cold. The capillaries open up and bring blood to the surface of the skin.

KAURIE KRIYA
Sit up straight, with the hands in Gyan Mudra. Inhale deeply and in a single breath chant:

SA RE GA MA PA DHA NEE
SA TA NA MA RA MA DA SA
SA SAY SO HUNG

This mantra is chanted as in a normal major scale (DO RE MI FA...) Begin with a VERY low note to enable you to complete the nineteen components of this mantra.

Inhale deeply and repeat. One cycle takes about 15 seconds. This, Kriya can be practiced for any length of time.

Contained in this Kriya are mantras of the earth SA RE GA MA PA DHA NE SA; mantras of the ether SA TA NA MA and the Siri Gaitri mantra RA MA DHA SA SA SE SO HUNG. In ancient times, this kriya was practiced by large groups sitting under a single dome in concentric circles. A single person would sit in the middle and lead the chanting. Besides the effects of balancing the inflow and flow of energy, this kriya will make the glandular system secrete totally in the same way that it does on the 11th day of the new moon (a time of lunar fasting where no food or liquid is taken to potentiate the secretory process of the glands).

MANTRAS

Mantras the 10 Body way!

ADI MANTRA:
ONG NAMO GURU DEV NAMO

This mantra calls upon the Creator, the Divine Teacher inside every human being. It establishes a strong and clear connection to receive the highest guidance, energy and inspiration.

ADAYS TISAI ADAYS, AAD ANEEL ANAAD ANAAHAT, JUG JUG AYKO VAYS

A yogic greeting to that Reality, which is pure throughout all of time and space - the experience of Oneness. The knowledge of the universe and beyond will come to you without ever reading a book. This mantra initiates you into that knowledge which is within all. It is the yogi's humble opening up to the infinite. This mantra gives mastery over the First Body.

AD GURAY NAMEH, JUGAAD GURAY NAMEH, SAT GURAY NAMEH, SIRI GURU DAYVAY NAMEH

Mangala Charan Mantra - Before Starting a Yoga Set Chant this Mantra

Press the thumbs on the chest at the sternum. Inhale deeply and focus your concentration at the third eye and then chant:

Ad Guray: Guru which existed before creation
Nameh: I bow
Jugad Guray: Guru which is throughout all time
Sat Guray: Guru which is True
Siri: Great
Guru: that which transforms darkness to light
Devay: angelic, unseen
I bow to the primal wisdom, I bow to the wisdom true through the ages, I bow to the true wisdom, I bow to the great unseen wisdom.

This mantra links you with the eternal space of the "Shabad Guru". The Shabad Guru is the guiding principle in Kundalini

Yoga, it is not personal, it's an eternal vibratory frequency. It's Sat, true, it never changes.

Clears clouds of doubt and opens you to guidance and protection as it surrounds the magnetic field with protective light.

This mantra awakens all 10 Bodies when the hands are held in prayer pose.

ADI SHAKTI NAMO NAMO
I bow to the primal power
SARAB SHAKTI NAMO NAMO
I bow to the all encompassing Power and Energy
PRITAM BHAGWATI NAMO NAMO
I bow to that vessel through which creation manifests
KUNDALINI MATA SHAKTI NAMO NAMO
I bow to the creative aspect of the kundalini, the Divine Mother Power

This devotional mantra invokes the primary Creative Power, which manifest as the feminine.

It awakens the kundalini, which creates a strong aura and this will give you the experience of security.

AD SACH, JUGAD SACH, HAIBHAY SACH, NANAK HOSI BHAY SACH
Truth is - when it stays true at the beginning, throughout all ages, in this moment, and forever.

This mantra connects you deeply to your identity of Infinity, for mastery of the 2nd Body. This mantra moves all that is stuck.

AAP SAHAI HOA, SACHAY DA, SACHA DHOAA, HAR, HAR, HAR
My infinite light from within becomes my shield and this protects me.

Gives protection and mental balance, it allows you to neutralize whatever is pushing your buttons because it gives you access to your heart chakra, your neutral mind.

ANG SUNG WAHE GURU

I synchronize my light with the infinite light.

This mantra transforms thoughts that haunt you into a synchronization of your light with the light of the universe. This mantra is for mastery of the 6th body.

ARDAS BHAI AMAR DAS GURU, AMAR DAS GURU, ARDAS BHAI RAM DAS GURU, RAM DAS GURU, RAM DAS GURU, SACHEE, SAHEE

Ardas bhai is a "mantra prayer". Amar Das and Ram Das are the archetypes for the 3rd and 4th Bodies. When chanting this mantra while visualizing a positive outcome and releasing that intention to your own neutral mind, you ensure that your intention manifests.

AJAI ALAI, ABHAI, ABAI
Invinsible, Indestructible, Fearless, Everywhere
ABHOO AJOO ANAAS AKAAS
Unborn, Forever, Indestructible, Within Everything
AGAUNJ, ABHUNJ, ALUKH, ABHUKH
invinsible, Indivisible, Invisible, Free from wants
AKAL, DYAL, ALAYK, ABYAKH
Immortal, Kind, Unimaginable, Formless
ANAM, AKAM, AGAAHA, ADHAAHAA
Unnameable, Free from desires, Unfathomable, Unbreakable
ANAATAAY, PARMAATAY, AJUNI, AMUNI
Without a Master, Destroyer of all, Beyond Birth and Death, Beyond Silence
NA RAGAY, NA RUNGAY, NA ROOPAY, NA RAYKAY
More then love itself, Beyond all colors, Formless, Beyond Chakras
AKARAMUNG, ABHARMUNG, AGANJAY, ALAYKHAY
Beyond karma, Beyond doubt, Beyond Battles, Unimaginable

By chanting this mantra you become the master of your own radiant body, then your divine shield will protect you so you can manifest your purest potential.

CHATTR CHAKKR VARTEE CHATTR CHAKKR BHUGATAY
Pervading in all 4 directions, enjoyer in all 4 directions
SUYAMBHAV SUBHANG SARAB DAA SARAB JUGATAY
Self illumined united with all
DUKAALANG PRANAASEE DAYAALANG SAROOPAY
Destroyer of bad times, embodiment of mercy
SADA UNG SUNGAY ABHANGANG BIBHOOTAY
Ever with in us, everlasting giver of un-destroyable power.

This mantra gives sahibi – control over your domain – self command and self grace and mastery over the 10th Body.

EK ONG KAR SAT GUR PRASAD SAT GUR PRASAD EK ONG KAR
One spirit beyond moves within the Creation.

This mantra needs to be chanted with reverence as it puts you instantly in your neutral mind.

Ek Ong Kar, Sat Nam, Karta Purk, Nirbhao, Nirvair, Akal Moorat, Ajuni, Saibhang, Guruprasad, Jap, Ad Sach, Jugad Sach, Haibi Sach, Nanak Hosi Bi Sach
I am at one with the creator, my true identity is infinity, it is that identity which accomplishes everything in my existence. My higher self-identity is fearless and without revenge. I am beyond death and the light in me existed before and after birth. This Truth is the formula that gives me that realization. The true light has always been, always will be, and Nanak confirms that this is the potential of all human beings.

This mantra lets us recognize our oneness with the true light of the universe and to relax because that synchronicity will bring everything to us. This mantra gives you mastery over all 10 bodies.

EK ONG KAR SAT NAM SIRI WAHE GURU
One spirit beyond moves within the creation this is our true identity, the ecstasy of this experience is beyond words.

This mantra lets us recognize our oneness with the true light of the universe and to relax because that synchronicity will bring everything to us. This mantra gives you mastery over all 10 bodies. You will be creative, connected, full of hope, a yogi, a teacher, focused, self contained, fearless and the master of your own radiance Unto Infinity.

GOBINDAY, MUKANDAY, UDARAY, APARAY, HARIANG, KARIANG, NIRNAMAY, AKAMAY
Sustaining, Liberating, Enlightening, Infinite, Destroying, Creating, Nameless, Desireless

For mastery of the 10th Body, it gives self-command and self-radiance for protection and unity with the light of the universe.

GURU GURU WAHE GURU GURU RAM DAS GURU
Darkness to light, the balance of Ra sun and the moon Ma.

I bow to the neutrality of the human heart, the neutral mind.

HAR Creative Infinity.

This mantra calibrates you to the expanding, rejuvenating aspect of creation, it heals the heart, the neutral mind.

HARI *Creation in action.*

When you want to manifest, and you need to be neutral, it gives you the ability for action directed from your heart, your neutral mind.

HAR HARAY HARI, WAHE GURU

I am in bliss because all of the karmic pain in my heart has been neutralized and I clear past, present and future pain. I am in ecstasy because I know how to do that.
HAR HAR MUKANDAY

Creative aspect of manifestation, liberating.
Masters the 8th body and will make you fearless.

224

HAR HAR WAHE GURU
Creative aspect of manifestation, bliss.

This creates balance between earth and ether and restores equilibrium, eliminates mother/father phobias. It gives mastery over the neutral mind.

HAR HAR HAR HAR GOBINDAY,
HAR HAR HAR HAR MUKANDAY
HAR HAR HAR HAR UDARAY,
HAR HAR HAR HAR APARAY
HAR HAR HAR HAR HARIANG,
HAR HAR HAR HAR KARIANG
HAR HAR HAR HAR NIRNAMAY,
HAR HAR HAR HAR AKAMAY

Fixes the mind on prosperity and power. It contains the 8 facets of self. You are empowering your own radiance.

HEALTHY AM I, HAPPY AM I, HOLY AM I

A positive affirmation for the 3rd Body.

HUMEE HUM BRAHM HUM
We are we, we are God.

Fixes the identity into its true reality, gives mastery of the 5th Body, creates balance and self-mastery as a teacher.

HUMEE HUM TUMEE TUM WAHE GURU I AM THINE IN MINE MYSELF WAHE GURU

Mastery of the 6th body, creates synchronicity between your light and the infinite light of the universe.

ONG NAMO GURU DEV NAMO
I bow to the vibratory frequency of existence, I bow to that which guides me to higher self-recognition.

Mastery of the 6th Body It is used to tune in before a yoga class, to allow for the student to connect to the teachings and not to the personality of the teacher.

ONG ONG LAKSHMAN

Mantra to connect you to the aspect of devotion, and prosperity. Mastery of 4th and 6th bodies.

ONG SOHUNG
I am creative infinity

Stimulates and opens the heart chakra, 4th body mastery.

PAVAN PAVAN PAVAN PAVAN
PAR PARA PAVAN GURU
PAVAN GURU WAHE GURU,
WAHE GURU PAVAN GURU
Pavan is the carrier of prana the life force.

This mantra increases the pranic energy and gives the experience of "may the force be with you" making you fearless, as it gives you mastery of the 8th body.

RA MA DA SA SA SAY SO HUNG
Sun, moon, earth, impersonal infinity, totality of infinity

The 8 sounds stimulate the flow of the kundalini in the central channel of the spine for healing. The ability to neutralize yourself and others so that healing can manifest. Mantra to master the 4th body.

RA MA
Ra is sun and Ma is the moon

Bij mantra, seed sound.

SA RE SA SA SA RE SA SA
SA RE SA SA SARANG
HAR RAY HAR HAR HAR RAY HAR HAR
HAR RAY HAR HAR HARRANG

Mantra gives you the capacity for effective communication, helps you conquer the wisdom of the past, present and future. It brings peace and prosperity even if it wasn't in your destiny. For mastery of the 5th Body.

SAT NAM
True Identity

"Truth is your identity" SAT NAM Use it as a greeting, anytime, anywhere, anyplace. It is a bija mantra, and awakens the soul, balances the 5 elements and gives you your destiny. Mastery of 4th and 5th bodies.

SA TA NA MA

This mantra increases intuition, balances the hemispheres of the brain and creates a spiritual destiny for someone when there was none. For mastery of 4th and 5th bodies as you will bring the frequency of your heart into your speech.

THE SUNSHINE SONG
May the long time sun shine upon you
All love surround you
And the pure light within you
Guide your way on

WAH YANTEE KAR YANTEE, JAG DUT PATI,
ADAK IT WAHA, BRAHAMADAY,
TRAISHA GURU, IT WAHE GURU
Great macro-self, creative self, all that is creative through time, three aspects of manifestation Brahma, Vishnu, Mahesh, that is Wahe Guru.

This mantra gives mastery of your own radiance, the 9th and 10th bodies

WAHE GURU
I accept my darkness and my light as this process of integration is what makes me whole and affirms my humanity.

It gives mastery of the 6th body.

WAHE GURU WAHE GURU WAHE JIO
I celebrate my true identity as infinity.

Mastery of 6, 7, 8, 9, 10, 11 bodies.

NAULIES to activate the 8th body, the pranic body.

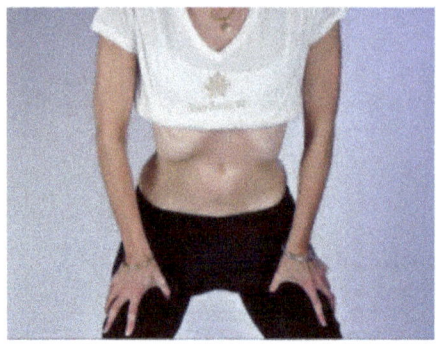

Naulies or Diaphragm Lock also known as Uddiyana Bandh: Energy and emotional control come from the pranic energy reservoir, which exists in the solar plexus. Naulie Kriya builds this pranic energy reservoir.

To master this bhanda we recommend that you include the following in your daily practice.

Do this only with absolutely no food or liquid in your stomach.

Practice it first thing in the morning after your cold shower and while standing in front of a mirror.

1. Place the hands on the thighs while bending forward slightly (30°).
2. Exhale the breath out and do not allow any breath to come back into the lungs while applying the bhanda.
3. With the breath held out, pull the abdominal muscles in and up.
4. Look in the mirror to make sure that the muscles of the diaphragm pull up, and in, and then also pull up under the rib cage.
5. Repeat holding and releasing the lock on the exhale several times.
6. Then inhale, again exhale and continue to apply this bhanda.

The key to be able to do this is to apply pressure downwards with the hands.

NUMEROLOGY READING

Yogic Numerology calculates five numbers from your birth date that illuminate your relationship with self, others, and destiny.

The SOUL number is the core of your identity. It indicates your own internal relationship with yourself—with the infinite, unlimited part of yourself. It is the key to tapping into your creativity and depth.

The KARMA number indicates the nature of your relationships with other people. This number describes the thing you must break through in order to be successful in your relationships with others. It is your "test" in life, which you have brought along with you many lifetimes.

The GIFT number describes your God-given talent. You don't have to work for it; it's already here and yours. You simply need to accept it.

The DESTINY number indicates the main trait that you have worked on for many lifetimes, that you mastered through personal sacrifice and effort. You may not see this mastery in yourself, but in actuality, it shows in everything you do. The destiny number is also a description of how other people see you.

The PATH number is the key to living a fulfilled life by understanding who you are and why you are here on this planet at this time. In order for you to feel fulfilled and successful, your path is the single trait that you must manifest in your day-to-day life. Otherwise you will always feel that "something is missing" from your life. Live your path and all else will work out naturally.

How to Calculate the Numbers

To calculate your own (or someone else's) numbers, use the birth date: mm/dd/yyyy. Keep summing the numbers until they are reduced to between 1 and 11, equivalent to the ten bodies and eleven, the embodiment of all.

Soul Number: Sum of both day numbers (d+d).

Karma Number: Sum of both month numbers (m+m).

Gift Number: Sum of the decade (last two digits of the year) (y+y).

For example, the gift number for a birth year of 1975 is $7 + 5 = 12$: $1 + 2 = 3$.

Destiny Number: Sum of all four digits of the year (y+y+y+y).

Path Number: Sum of all the numbers in your birth date (m+m+d+d+y+y+y+y). -Note this number is equal to the sum of the Soul, Karma, and Destiny numbers.

Note:

It is very helpful to create an awareness about which Body is dominant for you, because that Body becomes the hub through which all the other Bodies rotate through like the spokes on a wheel.

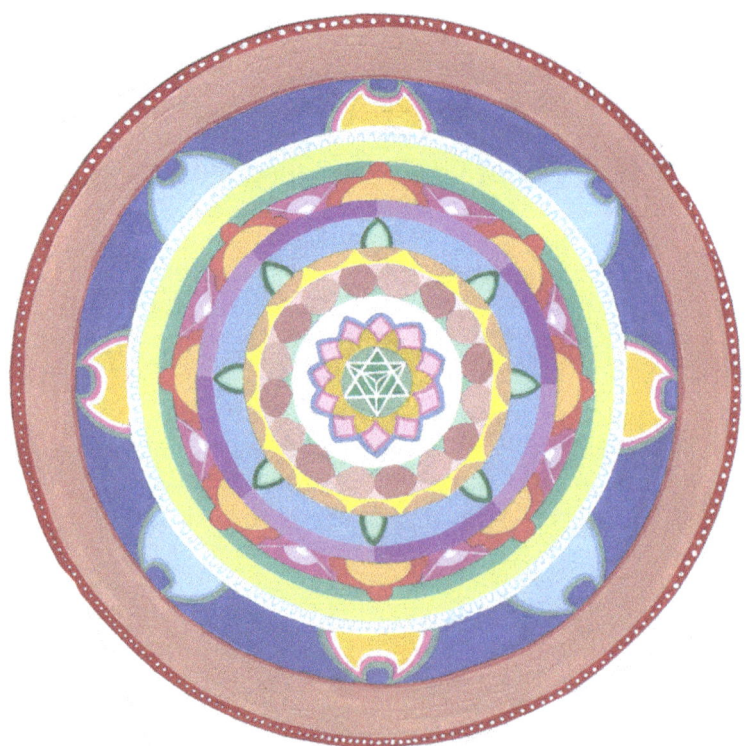

© Purest Potential

Self Mastery

Birthdate

month	day	year

SOUL	GIFT	PATH
day	last 2 of birth year	soul + karma + destiny

KARMA	DESTINY	
month	century	(example: 1964 10 + 64 + 83 8 + 3 = 11)

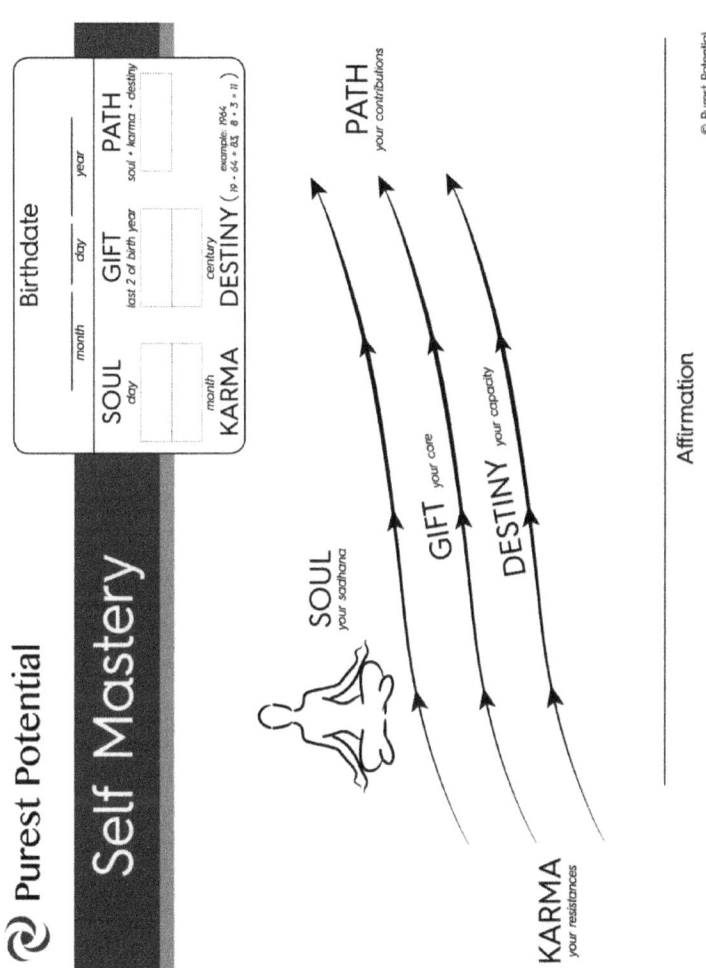

SOUL
your sadhana

KARMA
your resistances

GIFT your core

DESTINY your capacity

PATH
your contributions

Affirmation

GATKA An Indian style of stick fighting practiced with pranayama and powerful rhythmic movement.

Gatka Benefits:
- Gives the physical body a work out.
- Strengthens the radiant body.
- Creates royal courage in the psyche.
- Harmonizes all 10 bodies

GATKA - BASIC PAINTRA

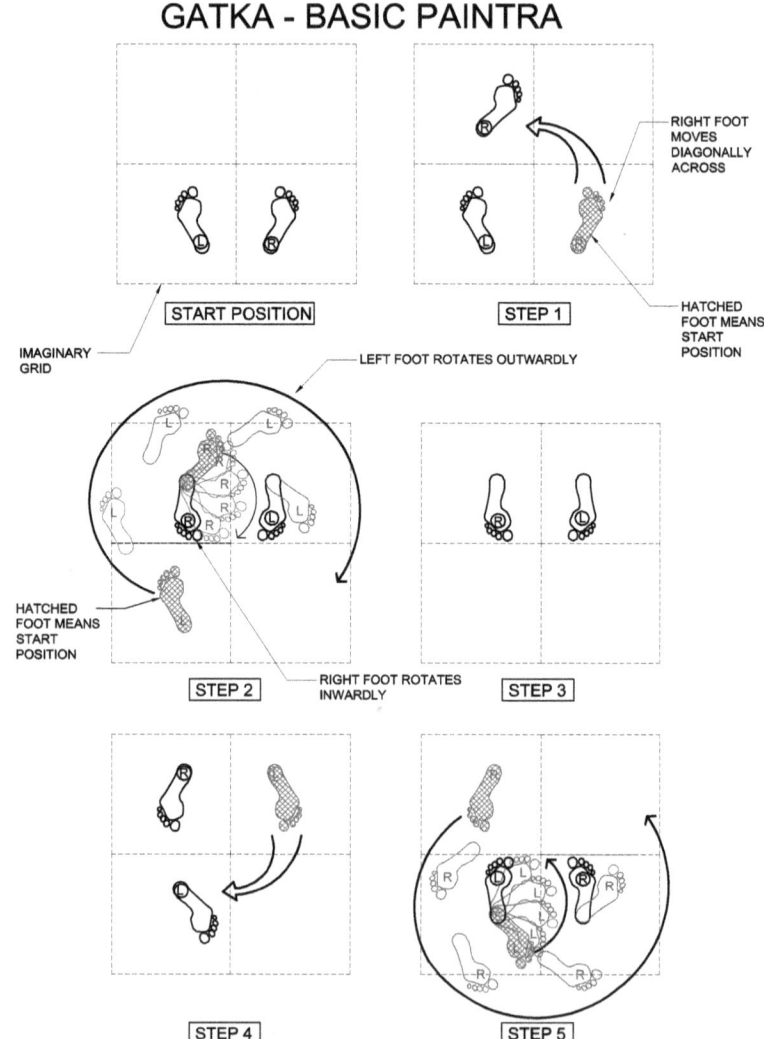

3 Step Transformation Process
Turn towards the Light

1) Pause and Listen deeply. Observe without judging those behaviors and conditions that are affecting me and express internal feelings states in a way that does not imply judgment, criticism, blame/punishment.

Meditation:
Drink a glass of water: place arms across chest, lock hands under the armpits with the palms open and against the body, raise shoulders up to ears, apply neck lock, close eyes, slow breath way down to 3 times per minute. **Continue for 3 to 11 min.**

Notice: What is my interlock, my reactive pattern/story?

2) Neutralize my reactivity by practicing Pratyahar (synchronize with Self)

Meditation:
Form a shallow cup of your hands in front of heart center. Place sides of hands together and point thumbs away from hands. Close eyes and look into palms through closed eyes. Chant *"Ek Ong Kar Sat GuruPrasad, Sat GurPrasad, Ek Ong Kar."* **Continue: 3 to 11 minutes.**

3) Turning towards the light, the joy, the awakening, to allow greater compassion, greater joy, greater connection to Source. Meditation for the 4th and 5th chakra: Apply Jallander Bandh (neck lock) chant *"Humi Hum Brahm Hum"* with the root of the tongue. **3 to 11 minutes.**

"See" your option of what response you would like to offer, then move forward and experience the joy as you transform your life.

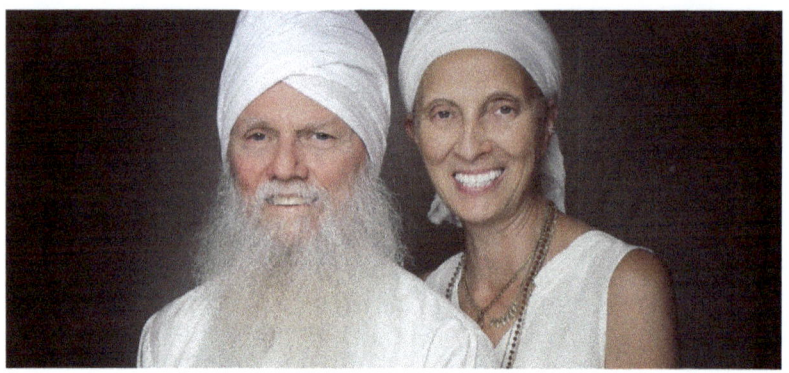

ABOUT THE AUTHORS

Dr. Guruchander was born and raised in Texas. He received his BA in Business Administration from Southern Methodist University in 1972, and his Doctor of Chiropractic degree from Pasadena College of Chiropractic in Pasadena, California, in 1982.

Dr. Guruchander began his study of Kundalini Yoga in 1972. In addition to his training in chiropractic, he has studied many forms of Oriental healing.

Kirn was born and raised in the Netherlands, Europe. She moved to the USA in 1975 when she was 15, where she was introduced to Kundalini Yoga. This powerful practice awakened her life-long passion to teach the possibility of living one's Purest Potential.

ONLINE COURSE:
Activate Your Purest Potential

Discover your potential and enjoy unstoppable motivation to clarify your intentions, experience deep inner calm and balance, carry through with your ideas and excel in your finances.

Learn 2 powerful yet simple methods to tap into your potential, so you can easily fine tune your physical world for more clarity, love, health, and wealth.

This is an evergreen course which means you can start it at any time, and once you purchase it you can access it forever.

The way this online course is designed allows it to become a safe space for deep listening, self reflection, real relationships, collaboration and co-creation, and to truly feel seen and heard.

The reality is that we live in a world where we desperately need more than information. We need each other. We need spaces that invite presence, deep listening, and meaningful connection. This is absolutely possible online, since we have the possibility to connect with people from all walks of life, all around the world. The work that you do in an intentional online community, can be a vehicle to create the world we all know is possible.

Out of deep listening we discover the stories which run our lives. This self awareness is arrived at by leaning into your stories and then to know in your bones that this is not who you are. You are not your reactions, your pain, other people's expectations, a to do list, or your accomplishments. You are so much more and you know this, deep within, you know this. This course is here to remind you, at times of forgetfulness.

Learn More & Find Out About Our Other Offerings at:
www.purestpotential.com

236

OUR BOOKS

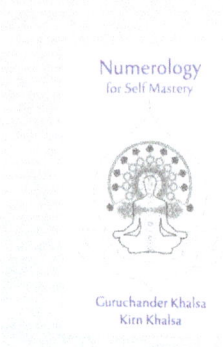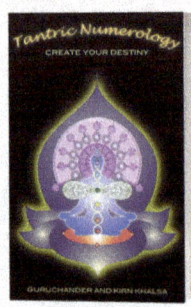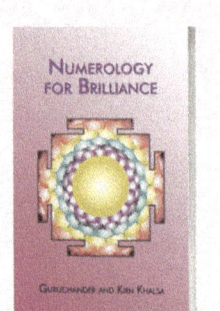

Numerology for Self Mastery and **Tantric Numerology** contain more meditations and yogic techniques to balance your ten bodies.

Available on www.purestpotential.com **& Amazon**

Would You Like To:

- Find a personal coach for Purushartha training?
- Schedule a numerology reading?
- Schedule a Yogic Energy Healing?

Email: **admin@purestpotential.com**

NOTES